Dr. D's Handbook for Men Over 40

D0971059

ISBN: 0-471-34787-6

Printed in the United States of America

10   9   8   7   6   5   4   3   2   1

Dr. D's Handbook for Men Over 40

■A Guide to Health, Fitness, Living, and Loving in the Prime of Life

Peter Dorsen, M.D.

John Wiley & Sons, Inc.

New York • Chichester • Weinheim • Brisbane • Singapore • Toronto

To Bria, Gabriella, Katarina, and Suzy.

This book could not have been done without your joy, questioning, and warmth. For this, I am forever grateful.

All my love, Dad/Peter

Contents

Many thanks to Leigh Pomeroy, a great friend and a master of understatement and wine, who helped make this book a reality.

This book is the apotheosis of people I have known since childhood. There were Rosie the Runner, Oscar Rand, George Ostler, Dr. Walter "Kip" Minaert, Al Merrill, Dartmouth Professor Edward Bradley, Seymour and Phyllis Lifschutz, M.D., Sylvan Moolten, M.D., Dr. Herb Brody, and cousin Norman Dorsen, Dan Tartaglia M.D., Paul Sandler, Norm Oakvik, Roy Carlsted, Arvid Krogsven, Andy McGinn, M.D., Arthur Leon, M.D., Michael Sprafka, Ph.D., Bjorn Lasserud, Dan Danielson, Chuck Burton, M.D., Torbjorn Karlsen, and many others.

Refuting a myth I had believed in, the staff at Chronimed Publishing made converting my manuscript into a success an easy process. For this I owe immense thanks to Cheryl Kimball (Director of Publishing), David Enyeart (Production Artist), Lori Asplund (Publicity), and Claire Lewis (Production Manager), who helped me believe what I had produced still continued to have unquestionable merit.

Let us not forget those woods where, on one of my runs, I could make my muscles tighten. After all, most of the time it was just me and The Great Spirit, without whom this all might never have happened.

Foreword

■ by Jim Chase, editor and publisher
of *Cross Country Skier* magazine.

There is a condition that hits many of us around 40 or so. It's perhaps not as menacing as it sounds, but it can be annoying at the very least. And as they say, it isn't something you "catch"—it "catches" you! It's called a variety of things, but I'll simply term it "middle age."

Once upon a time, getting older wasn't such a problem. The life expectancy for a man was in his thirties somewhere, which meant that once he lost that half step to the woolly mammoth—well, let's just say that his midlife crisis suddenly became the least of his worries.

It's tempting (and not entirely inaccurate) to suggest that we men aren't living the lives for which we were designed. Though it may be stretching it a bit to sit naked in the woods beating tom-toms in the middle of the night in our search for meaning in our lives, it is true that many of our physical and emotional characteristics may still be somewhere in the middle-to-late Pleistocene. Thus we find that we're having to adapt hunter-gatherer fight-or-flight instincts to the boardroom and bedroom.

Many of the traits we instinctively value—strength, agility, physical endurance, the ability to strive and compete—are no longer directly adaptable to human interaction, in which consensus and accommodation are often the key. Trouble is, implementing such concepts can cause stress or a sense of imbalance when they fly in the face of our inbred instincts.

The Slippery Slope of Decline

The physical side of our lives now has its outlets in sports and other active pursuits. But as any 35-year-old linebacker can confirm, as we approach midlife—through our thirties, and certainly by our forties—the sad fact is we may have lost the vital half step that once kept us from being lunch for something bigger than we were. Now we may be plagued by aches, pains, angst, or other signs of aging. This underlines an inevitable and painful realization that we can no longer do all the things for which we were originally designed. It makes us uneasy.

Fortunately, such skills are no longer so necessary to our lives. Walking into the boss's office and slapping down a bleeding haunch of fresh buffalo just doesn't carry the same clout it once did. Unfortunately, this thought is not always comforting. As outdated as hunting skills may be, their loss may cause us some anxiety.

There are other, more immediate pitfalls, as we all know. Remember the first time some 23-year-old lovely called you "sir"? Is she talking to me?

Now think of our friend back in the Ice Age, 32 years old and no longer able to compete successfully for the most desirable breeding partners—can't support a family, you see. Weak legs. Might just as well try to arm wrestle a dire wolf.

Racing Against Rats

Not that recent pressures are any kinder. Our 40th birthday may also mark a point at which, traditionally, we are supposed to have made some mark on this world, set our course, and achieved a certain level in our profession and career. We are supposed to have made major steps toward becoming "our own bosses," or "our own men." Daniel Levinson, in *Seasons of a Man's Life*, writes that age 40 is the point when many of us feel the need to cut away our trusted mentors and depart on our own life's adventure. Such a transition may not often be so easy. Although not always necessary, the jump can be another of the pressures that our lives put on us.

Now we want to be the ones to call the shots. If a man has not yet successfully achieved sufficient status, he can experience plenty of anxiety. "What?" we think. "Already 40 and still running in the rat race?" This is an eighties kind of concept, but it is compelling nonetheless.

So we seek ways of finding our balance, of being given that unmistakable sign that we've "made it." In *Iron John,* Robert Bly suggests that in modern society, we no longer have the rituals that once punctuated our lives and marked our passage from one phase to another. He (and countless men's group advocates) suggests that we go back to the rituals of our past—to "beat the drum" as it were—and re-create primitive rites of passage. Thus the notion of sitting naked in the woods. The intent is to give back to our lives the sense of balance that our primitive ancestors presumably enjoyed.

Such a rite of passage is actually not as bizarre as it sounds. The idea is that historically, people's lives—men *and* women—were delineated by rituals to celebrate passage into the next phase. There were coming-of-age ceremonies, first-kill rituals, leadership investitures, what have you. With few exceptions (weddings or bar mitzvahs come to mind), such benchmarks of life have disappeared. Lacking them, as the theory goes, we constantly feel we're not moving forward. So we revert to old rituals.

The problem is that our world is not going to change back. We are never going to go back to hunting full-time for a living instead of working as a dentist. Similarly, we may have to accept that some of the standards we once held for ourselves must be discarded in favor of a more realistic view of the lives we actually lead. The ability to run nonstop from sunrise to sunset in pursuit of a wounded prey is not very useful to the average businessman. If it were, it would doubtless be included in the MBA curriculum.

Obviously, we should recognize that what we do for a living has changed totally over the years—and especially during the past two decades—and that we shouldn't be trapped into judging ourselves by outdated standards of achievement. That's an easy thing to say, until the inevitable moment when real life intrudes on our little fantasy.

That doesn't mean we're advocating forgetting what we were or are. We have to recognize that while the world has changed greatly over 40,000 years, the animal inside us, *Homo sapiens,* has not. We have to be willing to adapt some pretty archaic personal traits to our modern world, and to accept that some pretty outdated habits, many of which aren't strictly rational, may go a long way toward making us happy anyway. In other words, some accommodation has to be made for the hunter within us. So back we come to naked men hunkering down together in the woods around the fire.

Generally, whatever works for you is okay with us. If you get a renewed sense of personal place from midnight woodlands reenactments of the rites of passage of a more primitive age, then do it. Then again, we're told that painting your face blue and white and howling "Go Cowboys" from the upper deck of a football stadium can serve much the same purpose. Do that, too, if it makes you feel better.

There's another way.

There may be some more mundane (and easier) accommodations to the Wildman within, as Bly might put it, that are well within the grasp of most of us. And that is another thing this book is about.

Jogging—Not Killing Game

The animal within us still makes its demands. The ability to run after game, although no longer necessary for our survival, is still what we were built for. Our bodies were created to feel good if we treat them a certain way, and not so good if we neglect them in other ways. Our pulses can be jacked up once in a while or our hearts and lungs may become unhealthy. When we feel anxious or threatened, our bodies still secrete hormones that are intended to give us physical strength, speed, and endurance. These same hormones, if not worked through our systems vigorously, can start to consume us from the inside.

The fact is, if the boss walks in and lays a heap of stress on us, our best response, physically anyway, may be to go out and run around the block a few times. Whatever it takes.

A good workout is good for the soul as well as the body, and continuing to maintain a physical edge still gives us a feeling of wholeness and happiness. During exercise we even secrete endorphins, those internal drugs that give us a rush and a delightful feeling of well-being—proof that this is what we were made to do. Our bodies are built for activity. Activity and pleasure, for us, should go hand in hand. If we don't get our heart rate up once in a while, we may start feeling as if we'll never make it out of our chairs again.

So even if beating the drum doesn't do it for you, don't forgo the demands of the hunter. Our bodies really haven't changed.

The Physical Man

Kathy, a woman friend of mine, once summed up how some women view men and their physical problems. One day she was in the office, not feeling very well herself. As I listened from around the corner, another woman came in and sympathized with her plight. "Gosh, Kathy," she said, "you look ill. How bad do you feel?"

"Terrible," Kathy replied. "As bad as a man."

Man Versus Woman: An Awareness

Are men really such a bunch of whiners? One of the little-known facts of male-female relationships is that women often tend to regard us as wimps. Some women think we whine excessively and complain ad nauseam about minor problems.

I hate to say it, but it's kind of true. Just harken back to the seminal *Our Bodies, Ourselves.* For some reason, women have always been more in tune with their bodies than men. Women usually know what's happening to themselves and accept what they sense is nonfatal. They know, for example, that as bad as childbirth may feel, it will be over soon. Think about it—in all the frontier movies, whenever a woman is about to give birth, the women escort the men to the outer room where they're safely out of the way and can pace and smoke until they're presented with a spanking new child and a wife who is no longer screaming in pain. What a beautiful picture. The reality is there are few pains worse than childbirth. And there is usually a geyser of blood and a kid covered with goo when it finally decides the time is right to pop out.

We men are not all that useful in situations like that. We can be even less useful when , for some reason, it's our own health that's at stake. Dr. Dorsen will outline some of these situations in upcoming chapters. Maybe it's just that *Our Bodies, Ourselves,* the acclaimed Bible for the female body, was first published more than 20 years ago, whereas men have never really had anything like it yet.

The fact is that from boyhood, men go to the doctor kicking and screaming. Ours is a reputation of helplessness in health matters. Witness the classic cold remedy advertisement: the clueless husband submitting meekly to the ministrations of a knowledgeable wife.

There are reasons, of course, for male-female disparity here. A woman's physical heartiness can be attributed to her being the bearer of children, a process that is often painful in itself and usually has its share of attendant unpleasantness in the form of hormonal swings, menstrual cycles, or dysfunctional bleeding. Occasional monthly complaints aside, women seem to have the ability to take it all in stride.

During her life, a woman gets ample opportunity to gauge the state of her health. It's a conditioned thing. Women have come to accept dysfunctional bleeding, menopause, the pain of childbirth, the nuances of menses, and the threat of breast, cervical, or ovarian cancer, among countless other assorted inconveniences. If women agonized over every ache and pain, they'd all become basket cases. How many women do you know who faint at the sight of a little blood? They'd be fainting constantly. Yet plenty of men end up on the floor at the first sight of their own red stuff.

Ailments From Nowhere

We men don't have such a built-in checking system. Injuries and illnesses seem to come from nowhere, and we sometimes might lack an innate or even educated clue about what's going on inside our bodies. In other words, many of us can get a little nervous about new aches and pains.

We can be such a peculiar blend of macho and mush. In spite of the fact that we get very anxious about the state of our health, we are reluctant to do anything about it. It's not manly, you see, to be rushing back and forth to the doctor's office. Besides, it might constitute an admission that we're not what we once were. We'd rather worry.

So 40 can be a tough time for many of us. In the back of our minds, we're saying, "Oh, lord, there it goes, the beginning of the end." Which, of course, it may literally have been, back in the days when we made our livings dodging large woolly quadrupeds.

Speaking rationally, it's not the end yet. Things are seldom so drastic these days, unless you happen to have picked the wrong plane, tied a love knot in your parachute, or been at the right place at the right time with the wrong woman. But we know you're bound to worry, so in the next chapter, Dr. Dorsen will go into specifics on your chances of dropping from "the big one"—a fatal heart attack, also known as sudden death—or succumbing to any one of a number of other things we're worrying about these days. Such angst can really scare any of us spitless. Although our bodies are changing, most of the changes aren't as dire as we sometimes fear. Whew!

The Mental Man
Mental Changes of Aging

Mental anxiety takes many forms: depression, anxiety, mood swings, uncontrollable sexual passions, anger, alcoholism, and drug abuse. Mood swings of middle age can cause divorce, abrupt career changes, adoption of fad diets, oddball changes in your wardrobes, and the purchase of expensive "toys" ranging from exotic exercise equipment to gold pendants to sports cars. The adage "He who dies with the most toys, wins" takes on mythical significance for some men during this period.

Let's face it—it's the mental anguish we're here to address. If the physical changes of aging didn't cause anxiety, there'd be no purpose in ever talking about them. We'd endure them, and that would be that.

We're typically made more than a little uncomfortable by aging. We see our lives and bodies changing in so many ways we don't like. We may even feel that we're losing something fundamental about ourselves.

Unfortunately, there is no shortage of things to be anxious about. Changes to our bodies are certainly not the only important source of angst. Our careers, families, social situations, relationships, and ambitions are also powerful sources of emotional stress. Our forties are typically a time of stress and change, and the era in which we live doesn't help matters much.

At 40, we regard our loves and careers as entering a critical phase. Common wisdom, for example, suggests that for our long-term security, we must "make it" now. Once we reach our late forties and early fifties, we're in danger not only of losing our jobs but, if so, of never finding another, at least of the same caliber and pay scale.

A man approaching and passing 40 has different needs from someone in his late twenties. In those carefree early days, for example, we could work for an employer without feeling stifled. As Daniel Levinson suggests, a boss or senior worker could fill a mentor role in our lives, and we were young enough to appreciate the guidance without feeling that we were being belittled.

By 40, however, many men feel that they should be making their own way. Often, we will have the notion that it's time we call the shots and that we shouldn't be relying on the wisdom or experience of someone who once was our mentor. We tend to feel that our stature depends on our independence from outside assistance. In extreme cases, unfortunately, men may resist any help from others. Some of us won't even ask for directions if we are lost. Women regard this stubbornness as male ego, which is, of course, partly true. There is also a strain of harsh reality here.

The American workplace is still very much in the male mold. Interpersonal communication on the job still tends to assume a distinct winner-loser format. A man who is not strongly self-sufficient may be regarded as weak. His stature and future suffer accordingly. This macho posture is wasteful, certainly, and it also seems to be changing, especially as more women enter the work force.

I found a particularly good illustration of the differences between male and female interaction in the experience of Steve Gaskill, former head coach of the U.S. Cross Country Ski Team. He once taught at the Holderness Academy, a private school in New Hampshire. In that capacity, he found himself coaching girls' soccer.

As Steve relates the story, he had more girls coming out for soccer than he could accommodate on one team. So, he decided to form several squads. And an interesting thing happened.

Holderness had so many teams that in fact they spent more of their time playing one another than they did playing other schools. Steve found that the expected did not happen—one of the teams did not rise to the top and dominate the others, as surely would have happened in a boys' program. A team of boys would have delighted in grinding the others' noses in it!

On the contrary, when one team consistently beat the others, the girls would actually trade players to achieve parity. Girls, it seems, were more interested in having fun—everybody having fun—and maintaining friendships by accommodating, if necessary, than in just winning. I have run across some pretty competitive women, but on the average, women tend not to be so knee-jerk about the whole thing. They tend to define as some of their best friends those with whom they compete on a regular basis.

The Family Man
The Changing Role of the Women in Our Lives

As in the workplace, a man's role in the family is changing, too. This is due largely to the shifting role of women in society, but there are economic causes as well. Since the early seventies, the actual earning power of a primary wage earner in the average American family has decreased by nearly half. This has created the situation so many of us face: In order to maintain the standard of living we grew up with, we need two incomes per family.

The male role, which eventually evolved into that quintessential modern man, Ward Cleaver (strong, wise, always home by five o'clock for dinner), began naturally enough. Women involved themselves with childbearing and child rearing. Men, because of their greater physical size, speed, and strength, became the hunters and, later, the breadwinners.

That doesn't necessarily explain male dominance of human society, however. Very likely, this was an attempt by the male to use physical advantage to ensure paternal claim on the children for whom he was hunting. Let's face it—you always know who your mother is, but you know who your father is only because your mother told you.

Though the myth continues that some ancient societies were organized into a solidly matriarchal mold, the truth is that men still held the power even in matrilineal societies—that is, societies where birthright followed the mother's side of the family. Perhaps those societies were more egalitarian than later "developed" civilizations, but there is simply no evidence that a true matriarchy in the same mold as the now traditional patriarchy ever existed. Perhaps where this egalitarianism waned is when men began to claim their paternal rights, that is, *their* women and *their* children.

As a result, women were forced into a subordinate role, subject to the men who hunted for them and could easily overpower them physically. This relationship evolved as society evolved from agrarian to industrial, but the essentially patriarchal nature of male-female interaction in the family has only recently begun to change, and only in certain more "advanced" societies in the world.

It isn't hard to understand, then, that men could have an atavistic aversion to women's establishing equality. Not only does such sharing of power threaten some primeval and antiquated male role in the family, but some male minds believe that it may undermine the very future of the species.

What is worse (from a practical standpoint, at least) is that as control of the world seems to pass out of our hands to be shared by women, the duties expected of us have remained the same—to be the breadwinner, to get a good job, to be successful. This is particularly difficult as men and women compete with one another in the workplace. In some cases, husbands and wives compete with each other in the household in areas ranging from who has the best job and who makes the most money to who drives the kid to dance lessons and who takes out the garbage.

Unfortunately, these changes have stressed some men beyond reason. Though there are other causes, one consequence is a dangerous increase in violence against women. Men who feel impotent in society might victimize family members or even strangers—as in the hideous crime of rape—just to prove they still have power. Though we must hope that as the anxiety passes, the violence will subside, we also face the necessity to take firm action to stop it and to protect our wives, mothers, daughters, and sisters.

Such anxiety is, of course, bound to affect our relationships. We're not here to suggest that family values and monogamous relationships are things of the past, but there are a number of glaring trends that demand a reappraisal of how families and relationships exist in our society. Dealing with such trends is yet another of the problems that we can't avoid as we enter our forties.

Divorce

Once, to be cast out, or "divorced," from the family or clan was synony-mous with being dead. (Jean Auel used this notion in her *Clan of the Cave Bear,* but the idea seems to have been around for a long time.) Because ancient man (or woman) probably couldn't survive without family or clan, being cast out amounted to the same thing—death. It was, there-fore, virtually unthinkable that a person could survive separate from the family.

The change in that view was made possible by many factors, not least of which is the movement away from the hand-to-mouth, hunter-gath-erer society. We live in the Industrial Age. We now have surplus. We cul-tivate the trappings of surplus, such as pets and lawns. Pets began as animals that served a function, but they evolved into animals that were conspicuously kept for absolutely no purpose. Lawns began as farmland kept conspicuously fallow to show wealth.

We can now afford to break up the family because, in many cases, resources are sufficient to support both the outcast and the remnants of the family. The poor devil struggling under harsh alimony payments or the battered wife forced to turn to social services might disagree with this, but it's true that our relative affluence has made divorce financially feasi-ble. Divorce is now a modern luxury—the ability to dissolve relationships for whatever reason and move on.

Families, Children, and History

There is certainly no reason to lament the passing of a prehistoric family model that was far from idyllic. Children fared especially hard. They were often raised much like domestic animals—reared to adulthood if conve-nient and profitable but sacrificed, even sold, if necessary. If food was short, it was the hunters, those strongest or closest to the kill, who got fed first.

This sort of thing continued in one permutation or another until com-paratively recent times, as a quick reading of Charles Dickens will tell you. The degree of civilization of a society can be perceived in the way it treats its children. Parenthetically, this is also why so much alarm has been raised recently about the quality of our own society as more and more American children fall below the poverty line.

There is solid evidence to indicate that some ancient societies were physically brutal to women as well as children. (Did cavemen really win their mates by clubbing them over the head and dragging them off?) A man's basic advantage was his physical strength, and he would very likely meet challenges using physical prowess rather than more subtle methods. The strong, silent type indeed!

Unfortunately, there are some men who would advocate returning to the days when they had the "right" simply to bash a rebellious mate into submission. Fortunately, most of us would disagree. On the other hand, we must recognize that the basic premise of such behavior, even if it's not genetically determined (which it partially may be), has been culturally ingrained in one form or another for tens of thousands of years. The transfer to a true male-female egalitarian society will certainly take more than a generation, and some would argue that it may not happen at all. A new order—including new ways of relating to our mates—is a work in progress. Men are still feeling their way, still making mistakes, still suffering the attendant uncertainty and anxiety. Although women are increasingly and justifiably impatient with this, I would hope they can be persuaded to cut us some slack as long as they feel we are making an appropriate effort.

What's Ahead?

In this book, Dr. Dorsen makes several assumptions. First, he assumes that the recent changes in the role of women in society and the family, with the attendant alteration in the "new" way men and women relate to one another, are here to stay. A corollary is the assumption that we are never going back to the old ways.

Second, he assumes that neither man nor woman is inherently superior. There is no magical feminine perspective that, once adopted by enlightened men, can lead to Utopia. Nor does he suggest that men are the misunderstood victims of rampant societal overhaul. Somehow the notion of men as downtrodden, especially after all the advantages we have enjoyed over the years, is difficult to accept.

We all bring something to the party, and the proper course is a liberal borrowing from the best in all of us. For our part, let us accept that male competitiveness has built much of value.

Physical Aspects of Change

The first part of this book will deal with the physical things that are happening to us. In the process, Dr. D separates a lot of myth from fact, so that you can come away with a more accurate (and, I hope, more comforting) view of what's in store for you in the next decade or so.

Next he tells you what to do about it. Here he stresses that the secret of our success as the human animal is adaptiveness. Yes, we try to control our environment and the circumstances surrounding our lives. But if the changes we have brought to our lives have made them more uncomfortable, we can take consolation in the fact that our very success at change suggests we also possess an uncanny ability to adapt ourselves in positive as well as negative ways.

Mental Aspects of Change

Also in this book Dr. Dorsen deals with what's going on inside the male head. (Unless your name is Zaphod Beeblebrox, the itinerant time traveler and certifiable male egotist in Douglas Adams's *The Hitchhiker's Guide to the Galaxy* series—in which case it's "heads.") Dr. D makes the irrefutable argument that the aging male doesn't have to fall apart and give up. The American male *can* learn to deal comfortably and successfully with the mental and emotional stresses attendant to change.

As Darwin might have said, we must adapt or die. Fortunately, that plays to our strength, because adaptation and change are what link our sub-human Pleistocene ancestor to our new man of the twenty-first century.

Preface

There were several reasons why this book happened. One was the sympathetic observations of several women in my life. They commented that a lot of my medicine columns in the latter part of the eighties in *The Main Event: A Sports Journal for Physicians* and then from 1995 to the present in *Cross Country Skier* magazine had a lot to do with my own personal struggle— getting and staying fit, trying my hand at high-level cross-country ski racing, worries about my body as it was aging, and sometimes fears of sudden death. After all, both my parents had developed first heart disease then cancer in their sixties and died.

I wrote about exercise-induced asthma, which I suffered from throughout the mid- and late eighties and spontaneously disappeared after I quit a problematic job. I watched an older Finnish racer drop and die during the 1992 World Cross Country Championships. Not only did his death make me question just who was at risk, but naturally I feared not a little for my own life. I knew I was redlining—going to the max. What were my risks in the 30K and 50K out there at Kincaid Park, Anchorage?

What was the difference between my participation in high-end racing and just regular exercise? What did I need to do to get motivated anywhere along the spectrum? That was how I ran across the "iceberg" personality, the *über*-athlete who could excel. What was the difference between going out for a fast walk in the woods and developing an anaerobic threshold somewhere near my VO_{max}?

Only after I decided to give up international cross-country ski racing did this book become more realistic. Now, my experiences could be readily available to anyone over 40. The idea that explaining ways of reversing the effects of aging might be helpful to someone who had not exercised since high school or college now seemed more of a challenge than entering a ski marathon. I began to think about these issues as I did my daily hike or run in the nearby woods. A lot about my upbringing, with its emphasis on athleticism, played a significant role in my interest. Between 1986 and 1990, during a self-styled sabbatical from general medical practice, I managed to publish numerous sports medicine articles, volunteer with Olympic teams, conduct sports medicine studies, and be elected a fellow in the American College of Sports Medicine. I also discovered that so much of what I was encountering in emergency rooms was not surprisingly different from the trauma of the playing fields. Likewise, internal medicine was an excellent vantage point from which to study both the normal and the abnormal in the human male machine.

My mother grew up in central Europe in the twenties and thirties, when Jews still had an equal opportunity to participate in all of the more popular sports. She learned skiing in the Sudetenland from her brother Howard, 10 years older and also a physician, her lifelong professional and personal role model. She and my father, before he contracted polio and became confined to a wheelchair for the rest of his life, instilled in me an excitement for skiing by carrying me on the back of their own skis while sliding on a small hill with a rope tow in Peapack, New Jersey.

As a result, I dreamed of skiing way before I became possessed by the mysteries of women, and I would soon find lots of opportunities to make skiing my escape and centering device. There were also swimming, diving, hiking, baseball, and football.

Throughout high school, I would ski bum in Vermont whenever I could find a way to get there. A family friend had his own resort, where I usually had the whole hill to myself, skiing untracked snow. Later, at Dartmouth, I had the opportunity to ski every afternoon of the winter, at least in my freshman year. (Alas, this led to poor grades, though I amassed thousands of miles on my skis.) I will never forget following our Austrian ski instructor, Walter, down the slopes right at the edge of the envelope. A characteristic cigar dangling from his mouth, Walter would schuss down beside us, shouting, "Okay, boys. Let's ze gut form, ya, ya, ya."

Discovering that Dartmouth had U.S. Cross Country Ski Team Olympic coach Al Merrill convinced me to switch from Alpine to cross-country. Thus I exchanged painful holes in my shins from high, stiff Alpine boots for billowy light Nordic canvas knickers, a pullover, and soft leather boots. The switch early on from the soon-to-be plastic world of downhill would be far more meditative for me. Everything about cross-country became a spiritual romance—nuking pine tar onto the bottoms of wood skis, hiking nearby woods in the summer and fall, and learning how exciting being outdoors in the winter actually could be. I loved the team sauna, and most of all how wonderful it felt to be truly fit (again). My first year of drinking and partying had been debilitating.

Then there were all those years in my twenties when I pushed my body to the max, through plenty of ups and downs, as a card-carrying workaholic medical resident. Moving into my thirties, during my early years of practice and being on call at all hours of the day and night, I lost my fitness. The effort to counteract this brought me back to serious cross-country ski racing, many ski marathons, and national and world championships.

I will never forget helping win the gold medal as the second leg in the 3×10 relay at the Masters Cross Country Championships at Lake Placid in 1986. It took total dedication to accomplish what sounds like a rather small feat. Truly, all the glory of the two previous Lake Placid Winter Olympics seemed to suffuse my body as I fought to win my leg of the race. I still remember trading places through the first half of the contest with one competitor I thought for sure was in my age group (he was, in fact, older). He fell, however, as we began the final dramatic descent into the Olympic stadium. I felt no remorse as I soared past him to complete the middle 10K leg to help capture a national gold in the 40-to-45 category. Only one person (or team) can win.

This continued until my early fifties. All of these diversions began to prove antithetical to my committed relationship, as well as to my need to be more available to my three growing girls. Ultimately, these pressures made me (and my wife) decide that I should look for healthier ways of escape. This decision brought me back to exercise simply to stay fit and escape from my stress. She even bought me a set of used golf clubs, but to no avail: once an aerobic animal, always an aerobic animal.

Although having kids has taught me what love really is, I must confess, I am still driven to escape into my own world of cross-country skiing, in-line skating, running, or simply hiking in the woods. Yet I am well aware that today's economics require fathers to participate in the housework and child care. The antidote—consistent distracting rhythmic exercise—can be one way to deal with life's everyday pressures, whether at home or at work. Life *is* exercising and happily finding some higher power in the quiet strength of an oak grove or in the instinct of a startled deer loping away through the woods. Your experience could put you closer in touch with your own Great Spirit.

I look forward to sharing what I have learned. I hope to show by example how it has worked for me and can work for you.

Chapter 1

The Fear of Growing Older

■ Facts and Myths About Our Bodies

Nothing makes one old so quickly as the ever-present thought that one is growing older.

G. C. Lichtenberg, German physicist, philosopher, *Aphorisms*

Aging confuses us. Some of us find it scary. We can easily fall prey to super-stitions, unreasonable fears, or outright misconceptions. One response to our fear is to take the ostrich approach and ignore or deny the nasty subject of our aging as long as we can. But that approach may serve only to leave us more scared and perplexed by changes that will take place inevitably.

What are the things that concern us? You can probably come up with a list better than I can. But for now, do the following sound familiar?

1. Am I about to suddenly drop dead from a heart attack?
2. Do I already have cancer?
3. Why am I short of breath?
4. What's going wrong with my back?
5. Why do my joints hurt?
6. Have my arms become too short, or do I need glasses?
7. Is my hair thinning or merely migrating below my ears?
8. Is my hearing getting worse, or am I just not interested in what you're saying?
9. "I'm sorry, my dear. I swear this has never happened before." (Sure.)

Our first order of business, therefore, is to discuss some of these fears and put them into some kind of perspective. Just what are our risks of death, cancer, and physical impairments at this stage of our lives?

We can't alter the inescapable fact that you and all your buddies are aging. So it isn't just you. Aging brings changes—and yes, things will change. Such changes fall into three categories:

1. Changes that aren't really happening. (I'll call them superstitions about aging.)

2. Changes that can be reversed, such as poor physical shape, the condition of being overweight, and many sexual problems (see chapter 2).

3. Changes that you have to learn to live with. (I'll call them the realities of aging.)

First, you have to separate the real from the imagined. In other words, you must clean out the first category and file what you find there in either category 2 or category 3. Sometimes this takes time. Sometimes we don't know what's real and what's imagined. And sometimes what's imagined becomes real, or vice versa. This testifies more to the weakness or the strength of our minds, depending on how that elusive faculty (the mind) is employed. But this discussion moves into another realm to be discussed in later chapters (deterioration of the mind), so right here, let's just keep this simple: Essentially, try to eliminate everything in the first category. What's left are the real physical manifestations of aging, some of which are changeable, some of which are not.

ARRRRGGGH! THUMP! (Or: The Fear of Dropping Dead)

I begin, naturally enough, with a concern that creeps into the male mind with increasing frequency with age—the fear of sudden death.

Imagine this scenario: You feel a pain in your chest followed by more pain radiating down your arm. You figure it probably came from that fall you took on the tennis court or from shoveling all that snow in the driveway last night. After all, your muscle tone just isn't what it used to be.

But then your heart starts pounding. You wonder: Could this mean you have a real problem, or is the pain just making you nervous? Should you go to the doctor or wait, hopefully, for the pain to go away?

You could be one of those men who literally never go to the doctor. Is such a pattern learned? You remember the time when you were waiting with your mother in your doctor's waiting room replete with fish tank, weird fish, funny smell, and overused magazines. Your throat hurt. Your ears ached. You didn't even want to be in school instead.

Then this large, red-faced man wearing a white coat came brusquely in, a round mirror with a hole in the middle of it perched on his forehead, a rubber tubelike thing swinging from his neck. Before you even had a chance to be afraid, run, or grab for Mom, "Open your mouth," he said, and stuck a fat popsicle stick inside. "Say 'ahh,'" he added, confirming that he would not set a conversation record. All you really wanted to do was throw up. When he stuck this pointy thing inside your ear, you knew then and there he had been smoking his pipe. Did any of this make you feel any better?

The chest pain continues, and you tell yourself, It's just gas, right? Or a spasm of some sort. Certainly nothing serious. You rationalize that if you were really having a heart attack, you would have at least had some kind of warning....Right? Isn't that the way it works?

We've reached the age at which all of us have a painful memory or two to jar us—an old college buddy who dropped dead out jogging. Who can forget reading about the late Nelson Rockefeller, who apparently died while having sex, or seeing an obituary for a guy only five years older than yourself who just plain old dropped dead. Now you remember your great uncle Sam, who collapsed on his 44th birthday and never came back. All this is enough to make us legitimately fearful, though too often not fearful enough to do anything about it. You think, "I'll see if it happens again, then I'll take action." It seemed as if in most of the ER cases during my years of medicine residency at "The John"(Johns Hopkins) and later at Hennepin County Medical Center in Minneapolis, I was trying to determine whether one or another 40 year old was or wasn't truly having a heart attack.

Sudden death may possibly be more explainable once the facts are examined more closely. Here's the real picture of how much danger you're in at any given time. My hope is in fact to lessen your fear.

Under 40—At this youthful age, your greatest danger of dying suddenly could come from a congenital abnormality such as an absent left coronary artery (one that doesn't extend all the way down your demanding left ventricle). This is med-speak for existing heart problems that are most likely hereditary; that is, from a birth defect. This is how basketball player Pete Maravich died.

Over 40—If you're in this crowd, your risks begin to shift toward such factors as arteriosclerosis (arteriosclerotic plaques causing coronary artery narrowing) and away from such congenital malfunctions that could pose risks to the under-40 set. This is especially true if you happen to have certain risk factors such as parents with a family history of heart disease, or if you have high cholesterol, diabetes, hypertension, or if you've smoked in the past 10 years. (Note: That's four out of five you can stick in category 2—that is, risk factors you may have a chance of correcting.)

Changes of Heart

It's important to be aware of those changes that are inevitable. Your cardiac reserve (just how much your heart muscle has in reserve when you stress it physically) declines with age, but that does not necessarily affect cardiac fitness. That's a personal biological matter related more to whether you decide to exercise regularly. In fact, age does not adversely affect your heart's response to vigorous submaximal exercise if you have chosen to remain fit. Things are looking up, aren't they?

Today's message: If you're fit, there's no reason why you can't exercise vigorously. Even though you're getting older, exercise and a healthier lifestyle (decreasing your risk factors) should continue to be beneficial. Just take the appropriate precautions. (See the Stress Test on pages 6–7.)

That's not to say that many of us haven't heard of guys our age dropping dead totally without warning or explanation. It happens. But it happens so seldom that it's statistically not significant (that is, the numbers don't lead to any meaningful conclusions). I'm still one of those curious optimists who read the obituaries every day. I'm one of those weirdos who also try to figure out why an adolescent or 30 or 40 year old has made the papers. My point is that for the most part, there is no reason statistically for a 35 year old to get some ink.

Generally, if you don't plan to exercise too hard, or are one of those lucky few who are risk-factor negative—low cholesterol, good EKG, all four grandparents alive and vigorous in their nineties, are not a smoker and don't have diabetes or some combination of these—just begin exercising slowly and try to train with the assistance of a certified exercise specialist. Later in the book I'll suggest several variations of fitness regimens.

Rumor has it that as we age, everything we have shrinks except our noses. What a bummer!

Take heart—literally! This is one vital organ that actually gets larger as you age. Such "adaptive hypertrophy" (larger growth) is sometimes for the good, as in the case of an athlete's heart, or sometimes for the bad, as in the case of someone who has congestive heart failure, a condition in which your heart may begin to enlarge as it fails.

Raymond Harris, MD, of the Center for the Study of Aging in Albany, New York, explains that the size of your heart actually increases between the ages of 30 and 90, largely because of heavier fibrous tissue in the heart muscle and valves.

But your heart can be a perverse muscle. As it ages, it may actually be shrinking even while it expands—that is, gaining in physical size but losing the myocardial (heart) fibers that make for a vigorous, efficient heart squeeze. This means that the heart, though it may be enlarging, is not doing so by adding supple, efficient tissue. It may be maintaining output, but it's doing so at a price. Long range, if this goes on unaltered, you may have a losing situation.

What happens is that an enlarged heart can no longer pump blood efficiently, and dilated heart valves can no longer be as efficient in sending blood up and out through the aorta to your vital organs. Though it's a bit more complicated, essentially the heart continues to grow (hypertrophy) in order to compensate, thus creating a rather vicious cycle. It's getting bigger but unfortunately not more effective or better.

Through cardiac enlargement and increasing stroke volume, a compromised heart can actually maintain adequate cardiac output, a vital ingredient for maintaining blood pressure and perfusing vital organs such as the lungs, the liver, and the kidneys. In plain English, stretched or otherwise aged heart muscle can pump just as effectively and achieve the same results as a healthy heart, but it requires care and conditioning.

But there are other possible complications. Failure of the electrical conduction system of the heart can occur at the same time as deterioration of the fibrous tissue in your heart. Your heart valves can thicken or become more rigid. These are aging, or senescent, changes your heart is inevitably undergoing. They're why a robust Kirk Douglas, still very much in the prime of his life in his seventies, suddenly passed out from a conduction disorder. With a permanent pacemaker, Douglas was back on the track again. An octogenarian and retired eye surgeon I know keeps outliving his pacemakers. His wife's biggest problem is getting him in off the tractor or back from cross-country skiing or tennis near his summer home in the New York Catskills.

More Changes of Heart

Your doc hears a heart murmur and becomes concerned. What, you wonder, is this all about?

By the age of 40, you should already know that the term "heart murmur" is not very precise. It refers to a wide array of gurgles, sloshes, hiccups, and burps that a heart may make in the course of beating. Kids' hearts routinely engage in such behavior as they grow and change. These are so-called "functional" murmurs, which are not necessarily of the same significance size as the valve abnormality. Once they've been checked out and evaluated with an echocardiogram, there does not have to be any immediate concern.

In the case of a 40-year-old man, however, there are certain possibilities that should be considered. Calcium plaques deposited on your heart valves may well be the culprit if your doctor suddenly discovers a new heart murmur. Just how much circulatory compromise you experience or is demonstrated on the echo determines whether a particular murmur is significant. In extreme cases, medical and surgical intervention may be necessary.

Other parts of the body can play tricks on the heart. For example, as you age, receptors in your neck become less sensitive to lower levels of oxygen or higher levels of carbon dioxide in your blood. Normally the function of such receptors is to increase heart rate to compensate for either low oxygen or high carbon dioxide levels. There is a chance you will run lower oxygen levels or higher CO_2 levels, especially if you have been a smoker. These receptors switch from sensitivity to low O_2 to high CO_2 levels as you age.

Doctors expect diminishing maximal heart rates on the treadmill as you age. A good rule of thumb of what to expect for a maximum heart rate can be determined by subtracting your age from 220. If you're 25, your resulting maximum heart rate is 195. But if you're 45, that number decreases to 180. In other words, as you grow older your motor just can't rev up as high. Most doctors aim to "stress" you between 65 and 85 percent of your maximum heart rate, using the 220-minus-age formula. Factors such as arthritis, level of fitness, or even unconscious fears about the test itself can determine just how well you will perform on the treadmill.

Acute physical strain, stress, or irregular heartbeats (arrhythmia) can accelerate your heart rate as you age. A fast or irregularly beating heart not permitting adequate left ventricular filling during diastole could ultimately compromise the amount of oxygen available to the rest of your body. This means that insufficiently oxygenated blood could fill your ventricles before its journey to your brain or to your lungs. The outcome can all too often be worsening heart failure, further arrhythmias, and even sudden death. And that's pretty much where we began this discussion.

THE STRESS TEST

If you're over 40 and about to undergo a vigorous physical fitness regimen, you should be a stickler about reminding your personal doc to put you through a thorough stress test. There are two reasons for this: One is simply to assay the state of your health. The second, related to the first, is that a stress test can ease your mind about your cardiac health. Both reasons are so completely compelling that I have difficulty understanding why any man in this circumstance would hesitate to get one.

The only thing I can think of is "the wimp factor." Men are afraid that the test will find something. There's always that atavistic paranoia, originating in that first doctor's office replete with tongue depressors and shots, that this might hurt.

Please bear with me, and I will try to convince you otherwise.

So what if the doc does find something? Unfortunately, there are some doctors who will go out of their way to worsen your emotional state by making such comforting statements as "there is no such thing as a falsely positive stress test." Oh, great. Talk about reasons to run in the opposite direction. This doesn't necessarily mean that a positive finding is automatically dangerous. It means that your doctor must take any finding seriously. You should, too, at least until further tests give you a clean bill of health. I can think of one dear friend and patient, easily taller than six feet and once a not-too-shabby college water polo player for Stanford, who dropped dead apparently after falling off the toilet during a six A.M. bowel movement on his sailboat up in the Apostle Islands of Lake Superior. Why? The autopsy showed little, and death by arrhythmia was the easiest choice.

If the results of your stress test are abnormal, a subsequent workup can include other tests such as the noninvasive thallium (or echo stress) test.

There are alternatives, such as a bicycle stress test, if for some reason you can't run on a treadmill and undergo a routine treadmill stress exam. Such alternatives apply if you have some physical impairment such as a history of a stroke or rheumatoid or degenerative arthritis of the knees or hips.

Regrettably, there are situations that dictate a direct look at your coronaries. If this happens to be the case, your physician may elect to schedule you for an angiogram. It's in moments like these that you might swish you were living in someone else's body. As unpleasant as an angiogram can be, it's best to remember that you are in a completely safe and controlled environment, so almost any problem can be corrected instantaneously by your alert physician.

Now there are a few men who are irrationally frightened they could drop dead getting a stress test. To these I say, fear not! Out of 1,375 facilities surveyed with 500,000 tests performed there was only one fatality. In statistical terms, this doesn't even merit a footnote. The bottom line is, if the test is indicated, get it done!

And Now for a Word of Encouragement

The old saying "What can go wrong will go wrong" fortunately does not apply to the heart. As I pointed out earlier in this chapter, and as I will continue to remind you throughout this book, by staying fit you can, for the most part, ward off that heart disease bogeyman. I have run into many men who, owing to their genetic background, should have died in their fifties from heart failure but are still going strong in their seventies. Just because the genes happen to fit doesn't mean you have to wear 'em!

The Big C

If we were all being honest with ourselves, we'd admit that of all the potential killers of men at midlife (AIDS aside), cancer is the one that scares us the most. Death from cancer is reputed to be long and painful, sometimes, it seems, made worse by our own efforts to save ourselves. And the whole thing seems so unfair. Unlike heart disease, which often hits people whose lifestyles have caused them to "deserve it," cancer attacks randomly.

Does it?

Not if we take a look at some of the numbers as we compare cancers, especially with other big killers. Lung cancer kills more than any other form of malignancy. Overall, it exceeds breast cancer as the most common cancer-related death for either gender. And it can be largely, though not exclusively, self-inflicted (by smoking).

But if we're talking about a pure terror quotient, we have to recognize the differences among cancers. Some cancers have high rates of occurrence, but not of mortality. Skin cancer is an example. It has the highest rate of occurrence but is way, way down the list as a killer.

So what cancers pose the greatest risks to the over-40 male? And just how great are the risks?

Lung cancer, as we just said, is first. Colon cancer is probably second (behind breast cancer in the general population, but second as a killer of males). Third is prostate cancer.

Pass the Cigarettes, Please

Lung cancer is justifiably famous as a self-inflicted disease. It's true that the most reliable way of getting it is to smoke. There are other risk factors, however, some environmentally caused and some not. Radon gas in the basement can give you lung cancer, as can secondhand smoke. Certain jobs that expose workers to toxic fumes are also dangerous. These are theoretically preventable. But there are also non-environmentally caused cases, too—you know, the kind that just don't seem fair. Comedian Andy Kaufmann, who never smoked and lived, by all accounts, a pretty clean life, was one of the more famous victims of lung cancer.

Lung cancer is to be avoided. What shows up as a dark spot on an X ray can grow and metastasize if not removed. The mortality rate, especially if the cancer is not discovered early, is very high.

Yet the risk of contracting lung cancer without exposure to such environmental causes (like smoking) is pretty low. So if you are 10 years out from quitting smoking, certainly check your house for radon, avoid secondhand smoke, and get a chest X ray regularly; statistics show you ought to be able to dodge the lung cancer bullet.

The Case of the Bloody Stool

According to J. S. Billett and M. C. Castleden of the Department of Medicine for the Elderly, Leicester, England, the colon is the site of the second deadliest cancer and is the second most common site of all cancer after skin cancer. A malignancy in the colon can often start as a benign polyp but end with wild growth and tissue destruction—that's why your HMO should always be anxious to go mining for polyps after you turn 40.

Colon cancer also has a surprisingly dismal prognosis. Yet the gastrointestinal system is another of those areas where listening to your body counts. Surveillance is the only reason, really, to discuss the statistics for colo-rectal cancer. In 1984 this brand of potential death struck 130,000 Americans (odds of getting it: 1 in 2,000), killing 60,000 of them. Three-fourths of the cancers involved the distal end of the gastrointestinal tract, often within a finger's distance of the rectum. Additionally, three-fourths of colo-rectal cancers are within the reach of a relatively painless diagnostic test, flexible sigmoidoscopy, a procedure easily done in any doctor's office. The American College of Physicians recommends for men over 40 to include a "flex sig" in their physical exam, and, if they are over

40, three hemoccult slide samples of separate stool samples (the simplest test for hidden blood in bowel). This is another way of testing for colo-rectal cancer. Keep in mind that polyps with cancer in situ won't test positive for blood until frank blood or even obstruction develops.

One caveat: There are false positive tests for blood in stool. The rule is that anyone who has his stools tested for blood should eat a lot of roughage but no red meat or beets for three days before collecting the samples. Fortunately, 7 percent of all tumors detected by this testing are still readily operable. The dictum, as you will hear me say throughout this book, is "listen to your body." You should respond as calmly as you can but decisively to pain, bleeding, or unexplained weight loss.

There's no question what must be done if your physician first detects blood in your stool or subsequently polyps during a barium enema, an easy way to "run your bowel." If you have any polyps detected and removed by the sigmoidoscope or by colonoscopy, a fiber optic study that goes all the way to the appendix at the end of the colon, you should then have either an air-contrast barium enema or colonoscopy every one or two years. Keep in mind that for a colonoscopy, you will get drugs intra-venously that not only eliminate any pain but leave you amnesiac. Such a deal. A major consideration with colo-rectal cancer is that the chances of surviving metastatic colon cancer are grim. You want to catch it early and, hopefully, eliminate it completely before it ever spreads. Although 20 percent undergo partial remission, there is unfortunately little prolon-gation of life.

Another test to monitor for colon cancer recurrence is based on the fact that a blood test, Carcinoembryonic Antigen (CEA), is elevated in colon cancer. A simple blood test for CEA can be used to follow the course of resected colon cancer and to detect any recurrence three or six months after surgical excision.

THE SEVEN WARNING SIGNS OF CANCER

1. A change in bowel or bladder habit.

2. A sore that won't heal.

3. Unusual bleeding or discharge.

4. A thickening or lump in a breast—or anywhere, for that matter.

5. Indigestion or difficulty swallowing.

6. An obvious change in the size or color of a mole or wart.

7. A nagging cough, hoarseness, or coughing up blood.

So Why Does My Doctor Need to Do a Rectal Exam?

Prostate cancer, the number three killer, hits about 70,000 men a year (odds: 1 in 3,000) as the third leading cause of cancer death in men. Black men are at highest risk, a hint that high stress can contribute to the risks. Again, early detection is crucial because prognosis is closely linked to the stage at which the illness is diagnosed.

Watch for the warnings. Certain symptoms are very suspicious. These include frequent urination, incomplete emptying of the bladder, or even embarrassing overflow incontinence.

Men over 40 should be tested for prostate cancer at least once every two years; over 60, once a year. Who wants to end up like Frank Zappa anyway? His prostate cancer had already spread. Make sure your examiner gets a substantial feel of your prostate for any lumps and bumps. He or she should draw a "male pap" blood test (PSA—prostate specific antigen), preferably before the gland has been squeezed, aroused, or obstructed. In case you were wondering, recent sexual activity can produce a false elevation in the PSA. Until recently some insurance companies have been reluctant to reimburse for this examination.

Data show that any type of prostate cancer with only a few so-called well-differentiated clusters will not increase the risk of death above that of the general population without cancer. But if the disease evolves to diffuse cancer at prostatectomy (stage A2), you definitely face a higher risk of relapse and death if the cancer is not treated.

Stage B, treated like stage A2, means a localized cancer is palpable on rectal examination, and you are a candidate for either surgery or irradiation. Radical prostatectomy, however, has a number of unpleasant complications, including impotence and retrograde or backward ejaculation, sometimes even with incontinence. Irradiation, therefore, may just be easier on your system. Men who have stages C and D prostate cancer, which means the cancer cells are spreading (metastasizing), are candidates for irradiation (for local control) or hormonal treatment (for painful metastatic bone pain, unfortunately all too common for those with prostate cancer).

Recent studies conducted at Harvard Medical School suggest a strong link between prostate cancer and eating fatty red meat. A high-red-meat diet is said to increase the risk of prostate cancer by two or three times.

Other Cancers

There are plenty of other less common cancers to worry about, but fortunately, the odds of contracting any one of them are pretty low, though the odds increase as you age.

Stomach cancer, although reputedly on the wane in the United States, typically numbers 25,000 new cases a year. That's a 1 in 10,000 chance of getting it. Here's a cancer that may have significant environmental causes, including dietary exposure to nitrates common in cured meats such as bacon and sausage as well as other carcinogens. If you are unfortunate enough to learn you have it, the cancer is usually already in an advanced stage at the time of diagnosis. Small-cell carcinoma of the lung is another "bad actor" because at the time of diagnosis in the lung, the cancer has usually spread to the brain, bone, or liver.

Another of the baddies is pancreatic cancer. It comes by its grim reputation for good reason. Of the 25,000 people diagnosed with it in 1984—again, a 1 in 10,000 chance of getting it—95 percent were dead in three years. The five-year survival rate is 1 percent. Like stomach cancer, pancreatic cancer is too often already incurable by the time it is diagnosed. It usually goes unnoticed until you feel some vague, yet frequently painful, deep abdominal discomfort. Then, by the time you find it, it has spread everywhere deep in the abdomen. Only 5 to 15 percent of patients who undergo surgery for pancreatic cancer are alive in five years.

One fact we tend to forget is that men also get breast cancer—not to be confused with benign male breast swelling called gynecomastia, growth in your breasts from drugs, hormones, or during adolescence. Breast cancer in men is rare as hen's teeth, but plenty fatal if missed. Make sure your doc does a 360-degree exam of both of your nipples, as well as a routine exam of your testicles and rectum.

Testicular cancer, particularly a "germ-cell" tumor of the testis, actually has a rather low incidence—2.3 cases per 100,000 persons. Testicular cancer, like colon rectal cancer, is another form of the disease with a marker that normalizes after a favorable clinical response, meaning it can be followed by a relatively simple lab test. Treatment is generally castration (partial, if only one side is affected) followed by irradiation of the deep lymph nodes in the abdomen.

Fortunately, a stage 1 nonseminal germ-cell tumor of the testes responds well to surgery alone—that is, castration with a radical inguinal lymph node dissection up into the abdomen. The good news is that combination chemotherapy is capable of inducing a remission in as many as 80 percent of the patients who have a disseminated form of this particular cancer.

No conversation about the Big C can be complete without mentioning melanoma—to many a particularly frightening form of skin cancer. Although skin cancer, per se, is the most common kind of cancer, what prevents it from also being the most common killer is that melanoma, the truly dangerous variety of skin cancer, is relatively uncommon. But melanoma is on the rise. Increased solar radiation, ultraviolet light to be exact (especially if you are one of those fair-skinned Scandinavian types), accounts for age-adjusted death rates for melanoma of four to five times what they were 30 years ago.

As is the case with many other cancers, genetic predisposition is a factor. Further, the depth of a tumor has a great deal to do with its prognosis. Tumors of more than 4 millimeters in depth and through the dermis carry an 80 percent risk of metastasis to beyond the nearby lymph nodes. If you have a red-blue gnarly growth on the back of your neck, your back, your arms, your leg, or anywhere, go somewhere to have the best doctor look at it and, if necessary, remove it. A technique as simple as a punch biopsy is least invasive yet can effectively provide the essential information between an appropriate full excision or terminal spread.

You can also get one of the several "liquid" tumors, the leukemias, all having their own course and prognosis. Keep in mind that I had my own practice for 11 years and never once found a new leukemia. There are also the "solid" cancers involving the lymphatic system, which, on a good day, strains your blood of impurities. These include lymphoma or Hodgkin's disease. Among these there's a wide difference in prognosis. For example, a lymphoma with very bizarre differentiated cells offers a bleak prognosis. But this type of malignancy, in the hands of a good oncologist, can respond very favorably.

Multiple myeloma is an affliction of the line of plasma cells that are involved with the immune system. They are virulent despite favorable innovations in chemotherapy and more radical methods such as bone marrow transplantation. Of significance is that multiple myeloma begins to have its greatest incidence (3 in 100,000) in middle-aged men. Median survival is from one to four years, depending on the amount of tumor mass at the time of initial diagnosis. These kind of numbers are one of the reasons I did not go into oncology.

Don't Panic

What can you do about the Big C?

1. Watch for the signs, some of which I have indicated above. If your family has a history of cancer, be particularly vigilant.
2. Don't be afraid to have an abnormality on or in your body checked out. It seems to be the natural tendency of men to seek medical treatment—or pursue wellness treatment—less frequently than they should or compared with women. If something's not right, don't be macho and just ignore it.
3. Make sure you get a proper diagnosis. If you're not sure after visiting one health care professional, get a second opinion.
4. After you get all the facts about your particular problem and the recommended treatment, do what you're supposed to do and try to keep a good attitude. Believe it or not, keeping a positive attitude is one of the best medicines you can get. More on that later....

Other than that, don't panic. Numbers don't lie, and they suggest that maybe you ought to worry a bit less about cancer after adequate surveillance and more about your cholesterol level—something you may actually be able to control.

When you read the numbers, also keep in mind that these statistics are not cumulative. Your risk of colon rectal cancer has nothing to do with your risk of cancer of the pancreas. In other words, you do not add your 1 in 2,000 chance to your 1 in 25,000, throw in a few other cancers, and come up with something like a 250 in 1,000 chance of dying of cancer in the next six months. Chances are that even in the unlikely event that you do get cancer, you're only going to get one kind. So your maximum risk is really only 1 in 2,000 for the most common type. no matter what.

So here's the kicker: After going through the litany of cancers you can get by breathing the air, drinking the water, or choosing the wrong parents or locality in which you live, the simple process of the narrowing of your heart vessels is by far a greater, but simultaneously more avoidable, killer! Five million Americans have coronary artery disease, making it—not cancer—the leading cause of death in males over 35 and in all persons over 45. Nearly all excess mortality in men is due to coronary artery disease. Despite overall downward trends in cardiac mortality, there is still an increase in the annual incidence of heart disease between the ages of 40 and 65. So much for truly understanding the significance of the numbers for cancer compared with heart disease. Heart disease is still a plenty big killer.

I'm not suggesting that you stop being careful about the quality of air or water you breathe or drink. By all means, reduce your cancer risk where and when you can, because the odds are that once you reach a ripe old age, if heart disease doesn't finally take its toll, cancer will. I'll offer more helpful suggestions later on—especially on what to eat.

So quit smoking. Above all, reduce any cardiac risk factors you can control because that may be the most significant way you have to decrease your risk of dying earlier than you need to.

The Process Of Elimination: Or What Goes In, Comes Out

Here's another of the unmentionables of aging—dicey topics such as suffering from a "weak bladder" or having "a good bowel movement." Aren't these God-given rights?

Should we really have to stop drinking beer or coffee out of fear of having to urinate every five minutes? (Remember the old college saying: "You don't drink beer, you just rent it"?) How about them vegetables? Prunes, anyone? How about beans or dairy products? Why do some get ga-a-a-ss?

Kidney Pie

It's a fact: The size of your kidneys decreases as you age. Your kidney blood flow, as well as how efficiently your kidneys filter impurities from the blood, also declines. But because most people have plenty of margin, these aging changes don't have to be of major concern unless you (a) have preexisting kidney problems or (b) become really dried out (dehydrated) from vomiting, diarrhea, or excessive sweating. Usually your kidneys have sufficient extra function so that they can tolerate this aging process. They can decline yet still accomplish their job with room to spare. Your kidney function usually becomes a major concern only when you take drugs excreted exclusively by the kidneys.

Any problem of excessive urination can actually be due to incomplete bladder emptying, especially if your prostate gland has grown with age to the size of a ripe Florida grapefruit. One advantage to being a male is that throughout much of your life, you have far less of a tendency for urinary tract infections than do women. However, increased frequency of, or a burning sensation during, urination warrants having your urine and prostate checked to rule out an infection, obstruction, or enlarged prostate.

If you have any form of diabetes, which is easily detected through urine and blood tests, you could have trouble with frequency of urination. And don't forget that your perception of frequent urination can sometimes be a response to emotional stress. If you're conscious about your urination habits, you may feel as if you have to urinate more. Or you may simply be unconsciously drinking excessive amounts of fluids. In other words, don't drown your sorrows in a six-pack or a coffee cup.

Probably few of us have survived this long without having some inflammation of the urethra. This is nothing new—not age related at all! As a male, you are definitely susceptible to any infection your bed partner might have. It is very important that you get treatment just as readily as your partner if she has infection of any kind. Surprisingly, despite all the attention given to safe sex to protect from AIDS, there is still an unfortunate rise in the incidence of sexually transmitted diseases. Sorry to say this, gentlemen, but unprotected intercourse must be relegated to history. Rain hats for all! Just as "Let me just say one word, son, plastics" was the advice in *The Graduate,* the advice in our generation has become "Let me just say one word, son"—or daughter, for that matter—"...latex." Believe it, guys, unless you're damned sure about your partner, "no glove, no love."

The Infamous BM

A lady once asked me, "With men, why do bowel movements always lead to vowel movements?" It took me a while, but I realized that she was referring to the male tendency to make a noise sort of like an "ahh" or an "unhh" during the process of eliminating solid waste. Certainly, a preoccupation with this activity can take on importance beyond all reason as we get older. Although it's not likely to be as critical in your forties, future worries about BMs can bring about plenty of anticipatory stress.

There are some causes for concern. An unexplained anemia, for example, can indicate some pretty serious problems, and in such situations, a full workup is probably warranted. But the gastrointestinal complaints that most of us are likely to have may take other forms. They arrive as upsets, irregularity, and general distress.

As we get older, we find we have to alter our diets. Gradually as we age, we can't always tolerate the same indiscriminate variety of delicacies we once ate with youthful abandon. Some of us develop an intolerance to milk products, for example. We may experience a lactase deficiency, so drinking milk can be accompanied by diarrhea, or at the very least, gas. This is a genetic deficiency of an enzyme called lactase, secreted by our small intestine, that helps us digest milk. It is deficient among many Asians, blacks, and whites, in that order.

There has been much investigative work done on milk and other foods. It was discovered a decade ago, for example, that newborns have in their livers a large number of receptors to detect (and thus deal with) low-density lipoprotiens—whole milk is full of them. As adults, we have lost many or most of these receptors. In other words, our bodies lose capacity to deal with fats or milk as efficiently. Our bodies are very likely trying to tell us something, perhaps we don't need as much fat as babies.

Then, too, remember that the whole applecart can be upset by stress plus too many chili peppers. If you get the medical advice to "cool it" with certain foods, I'd take the advice. Such an admonition can keep you from a nasty surprise from your gut later that night... when it might be too late.

And as far as regularity is concerned, that's still a matter of diet. But these days (as I continue to remind you), stress can upset the whole program. Smoking, too, can introduce some pretty testy variables into the formula. For specifics on how this happens, see the appropriate sections in this chapter dealing with the stomach, small intestine, and large intestine.

The Fire Within

Speaking of chili peppers, why, as we grow older, do our insides speak to us so much more often after meals? (Perhaps "scream at us" is more like it.) Why do we get indigestion far more easily than we used to in our indestructible youth? Why are we more prone to a hot stomach instead of hot passion?

It's alimentary, My Dear Watson.

Heartburn is often called "the working man's heart attack," and if we were to take an imaginary trip from the top to the bottom of the alimentary canal, we might find that many of the problems leading to gastrointestinal distress are self-inflicted and therefore are curable. Starting at the top of the food tube at the esophagus, we first deal with such predisposing conditions as obesity, drugs, or the angle at which you sleep, all of which can produce gastroesophageal reflux, especially if a man has a hiatal hernia—a gap in the lower end where the esophagus passes though the diaphragm. In plain English, this means that acidic food from the stomach creeps upward into our esophagus, resulting in heartburn. The size of the opening in the diaphragm for the esophagus as it passes from the chest to the abdomen can also be congenitally enlarged, allowing part of the stomach to move up through the larger hole in the diaphragm into your thorax (chest) and thus leading to more heartburn.

Not only food and drink but smoking has profound effects in this area of the body. Smoking not only desensitizes our taste buds, robbing us of the enjoyment of the food we eat, but it adversely effects where the end of the esophagus enters the stomach and worsens our heartburn. Smoking means ingesting tars and other toxic substances that can also upset the homeostasis of our gastrointestinal system.

Moving down the food canal, we next deal with the many reasons why our stomachs are more sensitive, not least of which are the ever-present stressors of a complicated world. The real biggies are the onset of significant gastric illnesses such as peptic ulcers caused by hyperacidity and infection, which ultimately lead to pain, more significantly, bleeding and obstruction. True, you may well be more susceptible (heredity is a factor), but a lot of the story is in how you take care of yourself. Fortunately, there are now some pretty good whiz-bang medications that can reverse or heal ulcers quickly and easily, as long as they're not in too critical shape. So much again for early intervention. The best medicine, of course, is still prevention.

A walloping case of duodenitis from heartburn can be the consequence of too many steins of beer, three-martini lunches, skipped meals, or unending work pressures. Bile-tract problems (such as gallstones), usually reserved for a mother, wife, or sister, are also known to occur in men with a genetic predisposition. So much for the five F's characterizing the gallbladder sufferer: female, fat, fair, flatulent, and flaky. So just think *male*, fat, fair, flatulent, and flaky, lest I appear sexist.

Liver Ailments: The Real "French Disease"?

Leaving for the moment our delightful tour of ulcer country, we stop in the neighborhood of our largest internal organ, the liver. We often call liver complaints "French" because as anyone who has spent any time in France knows, the French complain of liver problems more often than

Americans complain about the government.

The liver serves a number of functions, acting mainly as a filter and purifier for the blood. It is also useful in the removal of many drugs from the system. For these reasons, if the liver is working at reduced capacity, the effects are likely to show up in a variety of ways.

As we age, the relative weight of the liver diminishes as a percentage of total body weight, in part because the liver becomes slightly smaller, and in part because as we gain weight, the liver does not also gain. On the other hand, the liver does age the same way as the rest of our bodies do. Unabused, it appears to function as effectively in old age as when we are young. Testimony to this is that a liver from someone over 80 years of age can still be successfully transplanted into a young person and function perfectly well. And there's more good news: the liver is one of those tissues in the body that can regrow, despite injury from substances such as alcohol.

This doesn't mean we should take this organ for granted. Liver ailments abound, especially cirrhosis and other environmentally caused diseases. As with all other parts of the body, go by an adapted golden rule: "Do unto your liver as you would have it do unto you."

Strictly Glandular

No discussion about a 40-year-old man can exclude a visit with the gland man (endocrinologist). Our body is a potpourri of endocrine (secreting inward like insulin from the pancreas) or exocrine (secreting outward from the pancreas like amylase or pancreozymin) glands. All physicians—especially general internists and endocrinologists—deal day in and day out with problems related to the glands.

Purposely sounding like a broken record, I remind you that the whole body is interrelated, but nowhere is this more true than in the endocrine system. Aging beyond 40 can take its toll on the interaction of all the hormones that are part of this system.

The glandular system depends on a series of positive or negative loops from target organs (e.g., the thyroid) back to control centers such as the so-called master gland, the pituitary, safely snuggled at the base of the skull. Various stressors can affect these loops, even causing them to go haywire, as in diabetes, hypothyroidism, or hyperthyroidism. The importance of this system cannot be overemphasized. Causes abound that can make the endocrine system go off-kilter, including drug use, alcohol abuse, stress, poor diet, poor physical conditioning, or obesity.

The Pancreas

The pancreas is, as we should know by now, the source of insulin, the enzyme that allows us to assimilate the sugars that fuel our muscles. This quiet little organ lying under the duodenum and the small bowel, embedded deep within the abdomen and under the stomach, can get really mad when it wants to. Such problems often crop up at midlife. When this happens, doctors call it "pancreatitis." One of the more common consequences of too many bouts of pancreatitis is insulin-dependent diabetes mellitus. Type 2 is quite different from Type 1 diabetes, which is hereditary and usually discovered at a much younger age. Type 2 diabetes should be suspected when an adult who is overweight and over 30 begins to experience excessive thirst, urinary frequency, excessive hunger, or inappropriate weight loss.

Typically, someone with Type 2 diabetes will have inadequate insulin—hence noninsulin-dependent diabetes mellitus (NIDDM)—rather than no insulin—as in type 1, and can run fairly high glucose levels. (Later I'll deal with ideal weight and appropriate diets to avoid this type of diabetes.) Estimates are that approximately 6 percent of the population 45 to 64 years of age have this disease. The percentage increases to 9 percent at age 75 and older.

There is a truckload of predisposing factors, ultimately funneling down to how well insulin-mediated glucose uptake functions at the skeletal muscle level. Unfortunately, a certain proportion of the population is genetically predisposed. But there are a number of simple things you can do to reduce or eliminate your likelihood of developing Type 2 diabetes:

1. **Maintain muscle mass.** The American College of Sports Medicine advocates three sessions a week of aerobic exercise and two of anaerobic resistance exercise.

2. **Control body weight.** I suggest that men aim for no more than a 10 to 20 percent increase over their weight at the end of high school.

3. **Pursue an acceptable level of physical activity in general.**

4. **Maintain a good diet.** The goal should be to fill up on nutritional calories rather than empty calories. Three squares with two healthy snacks is the ticket. (See chapter 9.)

Be aware that as we age, there are plenty of medications that could interfere with insulin performance. Culprits may include thiazide diuretics (water pills), beta-blockers (which may affect how we break down insulin from our liver and muscle cells), steroids and nonsteroidal antiinflammatories (Motrin, Indocin, and others), and various antidepressants. Be a cautious consumer of all medications, either prescription or over-the-counter. Drugs, as helpful as they are, can be a double-edged sword.

The Intestine (All Twenty-Something Feet of It)

Back in the alimentary canal, our little submarine snakes its way down into the small intestine, the site for some mighty important absorption functions. Here is where our body, after the mouth and stomach have mashed and dissolved our food into a somewhat easily assimilated soup, actually takes in the bulk of its important nutrients.

Changes are occurring here as well as we age. Villi, the tiny fingers reaching out into the intestinal cavity, become stubby, shorter, and wider. Here is where problems relating to B_{12}, fat, iron, glucose, and calcium absorption can occur.

You'll find that most of the digestive organs are dependent upon other organs in the body for enzymes or hormones to help them operate. Some of the problems of the small intestine are, in fact, caused elsewhere. Vitamin B_{12}, for example, doesn't go anywhere without the vital intrinsic factor released from a healthy stomach lining upstream. Fat requires lipase. Glucose must have insulin. Calcium relies on the parathyroid gland (PTH) for its absorption. And so it goes.

After the small intestine comes the large intestine, which habitually causes more of a stir for the aging man. It is, for example, the site of a troublesome ailment called diverticulitis.

Supposedly, changes in the large-bowel wall structure that lead to an increase in pressure within the gut can be a predisposing condition for the development of diverticuli, small pouches or sacs in the wall of the intestine. Although most frequently associated with older folks, diverticuli can also occur in those who are younger. When these pouches become inflamed and suddenly turn into diverticulitis, trouble unfolds. Diverticulosis, usually a condition related to the aging bowel, is the presence of little pouches extruding from the large colon. Once they become infected, they are also called diverticulitis. For the past quarter century, the recommendation for these problems has been the so-called high-residue diet.

The large intestine is also where your doctor goes mining for polyps. Polyps and their more ominous successor, large-bowel cancer, are of major concern to the well-being of the large bowel. The latter is something always to be suspected in any man over 30 who suddenly finds himself anemic with a low blood count (microcytic, meaning small red cells). Other symptoms include a change in bowel habit; for instance, you notice that the shape or size of your bowel movements has narrowed to the size of a pencil. Blood may show up around, within, before, or after a BM. A documented drop in hemoglobin also deserves a workup for malignancy in any 40-year-old man, even though it may just be hemmorhoids. Low hemoglobin in any man over 40 is a serious warning sign and should be explored until cancer is positively ruled out.

On the Surface: Our Largest Organ, the Skin

What about all that body surface area we take for granted? That is, until Fido snags an ankle in his choppers or we sail over the handlebars of our mountain bike at 22 miles per hour. I know I have, but thank Zeus, I was wearing a helmet. They don't say "boys will be boys" for nothing, and it's true that the greatest threat to our skins when we're young is probably our own testosterone. In our teens and twenties, the "dumb" factor takes off far more skin than any ailment. But that wrapping—our skin, our largest organ—can take its share of abuse. Barring extensive burning or blood loss, it's usually a problem that can be solved with a needle, thread, a bit of xylocaine, silvidene cream, or steri strips.

As we age, however—and especially these days, with the ozone layer thinning out—melanoma as well as basal and squamous-cell carcinomas become a real concern, especially among those of us who are fair skinned. The danger of these cancers increases with age, probably because of the simple length of accumulated exposure to sunlight over the years.

So it makes plenty of sense for any 40 year old who has the guts to see his doctor, strip down to the buff so that the doc can look, biopsy, or excise what he or she sees fit. Once the diagnosis has been made and the lesion removed, pay the extra nickel to have it sent to pathology rather than let the doctor throw it away. If it is malignant or premalignant, the current routine is to remove the little bugger completely, which means taking plenty of flesh around all sides (Shylock would love this) in order to leave the area totally free of cancer. Laser is rapidly becoming the fastest, most efficient, and least painful method of excision available.

Liver Spots

Is 40 too early to start worrying about these traditional, unmistakable signs of age? Not really. As a matter of fact, the forties are the perfect time—not to worry, really, but to become aware.

Liver spots, in fact, have nothing whatsoever to do with the liver, but rather are the results of photoaging. They can be lightened by laser or by being burned off, or they can prevented altogether with sunscreens. Once again, ozone loss has made selectively avoiding the sun and wearing sunscreens imperative. You may not be able to reverse whatever damage was done when you were fried at a family beach picnic as a youngster, but you can help the odds by being vigilant today.

And while you're protecting yourself, don't neglect to protect the children. There's no sense perpetuating the same mistakes your parents made with you on your own offspring—or anyone else's offspring, for that matter.

Quite a number of other skin problems can develop as we age, mostly minor. Some of us get "skin tags," especially around the neck and armpits. They are easily snipped off and cauterized. Papules on skin aged in the sun occur frequently; our only concern is that they may transform into cancer. Here's where some doctors like to take one or more "punch biopsies" of a suspicious-looking lesion. If it returns positive for the Big C, then a full, wide excision becomes imperative.

By now, we've all noticed that the bronze-god ski instructors we so envied in our youth now look old enough to be our parents. The sun may supply plenty of vitamin D, but photoaging of the skin is no joke. Doctors warn that prevention is clearly the most effective method to ward off both wrinkles and disease. Most dermatologists, as a matter of fact, think that it's pretty silly to want a suntan. It is important that during both childhood and adulthood we encourage the use of sunscreens (SPF15 or greater), avoid excessive sunbathing and all tanning salons, and, in particular, shun any exposure to sun during midday. The traditional siesta (in the shade, of course) in many of the world's hot climates may make even more health sense than we realized.

Herpes

Herpes, as our dating friends remind us, unfortunately remains the gift that keeps on giving. There is still no way of getting rid of it. The 40-year-old stud, suddenly divorced and thrashing around in his midlife second childhood, must be constantly on the lookout for the possibility of herpes hominis 1 or 2. The former resides predominantly in the mouth; the latter calls the genitalia (both male and female) home. Fortunately, at the onset of either form of herpes, one of two forms of acyclovir, an effective antiviral medication, can render a new attack less painful and shorter lived by hastening the herpes into the inactive form.

Herpes hominis should not be confused with herpes zoster, also known among the older set as shingles, which tends to choose a single nerve root and follow it painfully around on one side of the body. Especially uncomfortable in anyone who has contracted zoster is post-herpetic neuralgia, which is only sometimes responsive to several new medications such as Tegretol (an antiseizure drug) or, in the acute phase, Zostrix, a pepper cream made from capsaicin.

If you recall the seventies, herpes stood as the sexually transmitted "plague" of the decade. Little did we know that within a few years, AIDS would appear to give stark new meaning to that term. Herpes, though certainly to be avoided, has been revealed as a relatively benign nuisance except when it afflicts the eye along the trigeminal root, requiring opthamological intervention. Though nobody wants it, contracting herpes (fortunately) isn't the end of the world.

Miscellaneous Skin Problems

Other annoying, though usually benign, dermal afflictions that occur in the over-40 crowd include eczema, atopic dermatitis, and psoriasis, which causes itching and flaking of the scalp or other parts of the body but is usually responsive to topical steroids, tar-containing ointments, or light treatments. Then there is scabies, the troublesome little mite, and head lice, both of which can leap to 40-year-old daddy from junior who caught it at day care or school. Finally, you will find that plain old dry skin becomes problematic, particularly on the feet and hands. Here you'll have to try out a variety of topical ointments or creams to see what works on your skin. Don't hesitate to ask your pharmacist for advice. He or she often knows what works and what doesn't, and why.

ALCOHOL: "A GOOD FAMILIAR CREATURE IF IT BE WELL USED"

Alcohol is not an essential body fluid, although for some guys you would think so. Yet certainly no discussion of disease in men over 40 can exclude the stuff, said to be responsible for roughly 200,000 deaths in the United States every year. Reasons for alcohol abuse vary from mental and emotional stress to heredity. (We'll deal with many of them in upcoming chapters.) Either way, the effects are unmistakable—seizures ("rum fits"), hallucinations, delirium tremens (the "DT's"), nutritional disorders, and retrograde amnesia, not to mention increased odds of contracting cancer. Smoke and alcohol equals cancer of the mouth or of the lung.

Such outcomes are certainly bad enough, but perhaps there are also more insidious signs of abuse. A steady, far-less-than-toxic diet of alcohol can still alter personality (if you happen to have the right genes) and can also induce paranoia or aggression, interrupt sleep patterns, interfere with concentration and creativity, lead to mood disorders, and generally create a situation that can end jobs, break marriages, or destroy relationships. Because the afflicted one does not have to be a drop-down, staggering drunk, the disease can be that much harder to recognize.

I'm not one for total abstinence, because a glass of red wine (Oh, damn, I like a dry light white now and then) has proven beneficial to the heart and circulatory system. To quote the late Mr. Jay Phillips on his liquor bottles, "drink in moderation." Remember, each body is different: Some show the effects of alcohol more readily and, unfortunately, more erratically than others. Just because your buddy can drink a six-pack and play three rounds of tennis on a 90-degree day doesn't mean that you can. Listen to your body…and remember what William Shakespeare warned: "[Drink] provokes the desire, but it takes away the performance."

A Midlife Trip to the Dentist

OK, so going to the dentist may not rank as your favorite activity. We've all had our horrifying experiences to look back on, and such memories tend to make our trips to the tooth doctor rank somewhere below a tax audit, an afternoon in a storm cellar with your accountant, and a case of the flu. As we cruise past 40, the pain and gore are accompanied by an endless discourse from the dentist on what even more terrifying things are going to happen to our mouths if we don't floss and get cleaned more often.

According to Dr. Roger Bromaghin, DDS, a humble country dentist from Big Lake, Minnesota, you should pay heed.

As you age, your teeth generally become weaker and can fracture without much provocation (from lead shot, a popcorn kernel, a bit of bone, some hard candy, cough drops, etc.). In my own case, I had just spent several horrible days undergoing a root canal a year down the pike from major gum (periodontal) surgery, when my tooth fractured eating lasagna. As fillings laid in your youth begin to break down and their margins chip away, the filling-to-tooth interface widens, becoming an ideal location for decay and further weakening. Many of the plus-40 male crowd like me grew up in the era before dental floss was de rigueur, so this successful method for preventing gums from becoming infected, the habit of flossing at least at bedtime but preferably after all meals, is an acquired one—often with difficulty.

The major problem is that bacteria-producing foods such as carbohydrates are often retained in the mouth. What follows is that amylase in the saliva breaks down any starches (dried fruits, crackers, pretzels, potato chips) stuck between the teeth in those widening crevices where fillings have shrunk, allowing bacteria to have a field day. Not only do such bacteria cause cavities; they're why your wife may turn pale and dive under the pillow when you try to kiss her in the morning.

Periodontal Disease: Your Mouth's Number One Enemy

The number one problem for men over 40, however, is periodontal disease—the infection of the gums and supporting tissue of the teeth. The most common periodontal disease is periodontitis, an infection due to retained bacteria in plaque and cavities under the gums. Fortunately, this problem is largely preventable and can be corrected with good oral hygiene—brushing, flossing, and avoiding especially sticky sweet foods.

Dentists like to advocate flossing. You'd think they owned stock in dental floss futures or toothbrushes. (The latest, by the way, is dental floss made of Gore-Tex, the same stuff that forms the membrane in waterproof/breathable outerwear.) However, flossing once a day does remove plaque. The critical time for daily flossing is at bedtime, when salivary flow, which can bathe away bacteria, is at its lowest rate.

Smoking contributes to periodontal disease, making it both more severe and more widely distributed in the mouth. I know smokers who have lost teeth *without cavities* to periodontal disease. Smokeless tobacco changes gum tissue as well and when used with alcohol on a regular basis has been called an ideal medium for developing squamous carcinoma of the mouth—not exactly a pretty way to die. These are the guys who get half their gums or throat cut out.

Caffeine, fortunately, presents no more of a threat at this point than staining the teeth. Too much chewing or grinding (chewing tons of gum or unconscious grinding of your teeth while you sleep) can lead to serious pain on the temporomandibular joint. Culprits that can lead to TMJ pain include excessive gum chewing, nail biting, pipe smoking, or bruxing— bruxism is unconsciously grinding the jaw from side to side while you are sleeping. Teeth clenching caused by tension can create problems.

Sorry to say this, fellows, but your dentist is probably right: Virtually everyone over 40 has some degree of periodontal disease. We all live with it. Plaque at the gum line or just below the gum line provides the perfect medium for bacteria, which further loosen the gum and attack the softer part of the tooth normally protected by the gum. The trouble really becomes serious when periodontal disease works its way toward the apex of the tooth root. Plus, minerals from saliva alone can build up destructive tarter and calcification within just 24 hours. (I think dentists do own futures in dental floss.)

Can your teeth be saved? Yes, but good teeth and a resistance to periodontal disease take good genes—something you can't do much about. It is important to practice a significant, but routine, daily flossing effort, something you can do. I wish I could offer you an exotic and significant breakthrough for preventing periodontal disease at this point, but that just hasn't happened. Until then, it's a simple matter of brushing, flossing, stimulating the gums with a gum stimulator, and getting those pearly whites scraped every six months to a year.

Oh—and quit smoking!

A Final Word

The bottom line is this: There are two sides to the physical changes of aging. The first is that some of these changes are going to happen no matter what you do. The second is that just because you are aging and changing, there's no reason why it has to make you miserable.

The one mistake you really want to avoid is avoidance itself. Denying obvious symptoms, or failing to inform yourself about what's really happening to your body, will only make you prey to all the misinformation and myth surrounding the male aging process. Further, it will rob you of the opportunity of taking those steps that can blunt the sting of aging and add joy and happiness to the rest of your life.

That said, it's time to get into more detail.

SUGGESTED READINGS

Clayman, Charles. *The AMA Family Guide.* Random House, 1994. 880 pp.

Griffith, H. Winter, MD. *Complete Guide to Symptoms, Illness, and Surgery.* Body Press Peregen Books, 1995. 1,080 pp.

Hall, Marty. *One Stride Ahead.* Winchester Press, 1981. 242 pp.

Larson, David. *Mayo Clinic Family Health Book.* Morrow, 1996. 1,438 pp.

Obeck, Vic. *How to Exercise Without Moving a Muscle.* Pocket Books, 1964. 89 pp.

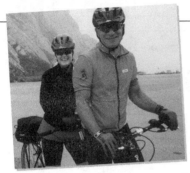

Barry Mink, MD

What's 100 Miles, More or Less?

Dr. Barry Mink's life has run the gamut from being a catcher for the Boston Red Sox to having an internal medicine practice in Aspen, Colorado. And now that he's 56, life is still taking twists and turns. For example, this soft-spoken physician who is built like a fire hydrant now runs marathons, bikes 100 miles at a shot, cross-country skis, and more.

"All my races are over 100 miles," he says. "I've done many marathons, but I discovered I couldn't win it in the fast lane, so I tackled races like the Leadville 100 for mountain bikes, which I've done three years now. I've promised my wife I wouldn't do it this year." But he adds with a wink, "Maybe I'll do the Cross-Country World Masters at Lake Placid instead."

Despite this intensity, Barry has learned to keep a balanced perspective. That's because in the past, he admits he may have been a bit too focused on his training, stealing time from both his practice and his family. Despite working hard to fit his training in during lunch or before or after work, he would invariably often be a little late. Patients would begin to question his professionalism, and his associates would grumble. Says Barry, "There was no question I was a good doctor, but this was just not the good old guy sitting there listening."

He confesses that he may also have neglected his three daughters a bit while they were growing up. "Thank God my wife was flexible," he says. "Certainly there are some aspects of my life I would have changed. Yet exercise is so important. Being the 'warrior athlete' relieves stress." Whatever he did must have worked, because the girls, now all grown up, are doing great, and his marriage is still going strong after 30 years, making him and his wife a rare breed in Aspen. Perhaps one reason for their success is that several years ago, he bought a tandem bicycle so he and his wife can tour locally or along the California coast.

Today Dr. Mink is as quick as any practicing physician to acknowledge that once you're over 50, maximal oxygen uptake and strength decline. But by improving the efficiency of technique, older males can remain competitive far beyond what age might dictate. "I exercise an hour a day, though sometimes my 35 to 60 minutes gets cut off due to work," he says. "On the weekend, I try to get in two to five hours, depending. But now I'm riding a tandem mountain bike with my wife. I guess no more lonely, long three to four hour runs for me. I'm excited."

Dr. Barry Mink is a fascinating set of paradoxes. He admits that life is "not without its risks, its bumps and bruises." Still, it's hard not to be impressed while sitting with him over dinner. Maybe that's because there have always been certain inviolate constants in his life: his medicine, his family, and his marriage. I guess that's why it's not difficult imagining Barry as a young man, the son of a Chicago physical education teacher, crouched behind home plate awaiting a 90 mile-per-hour fastball. Or seeing him today in the 99th mile of a 100-mile mountain bike race, he's just as eager as when he began at the starting line.

Chapter 2

Physical Changes
That Affect
Physical Ability

The years between fifty and seventy are the hardest. You are always being asked to do things, and yet you are not decrepit enough to turn them down.

T. S. Eliot, *Time,* Oct. 23, 1950

As you get older, you should inevitably expect to see a lessening in what you might expect of yourself physically. Realistically, what you have intellectually and physically won't be as strong or as quick; your endurance will no longer be boundless. If this weren't true, the average football career wouldn't end by the time a player hits 35.

Though no one has discovered the whereabouts yet of an eternal fountain of youth, the upbeat news is that there are always going to be legitimate ways to delay or just compensate for the aging process and even prevent some of the often-considered inevitable consequences of aging— e.g., a reduced cardiac output or just how fast we can run on a track or swim in a pool. In chapter 1, I covered many (but certainly not all) of the physical changes the male body undergoes as it ages. What follows in this chapter is an overview of some of the key changes that affect the male body in its drive to run faster and jump higher, and what inevitably becomes the challenge of at least keeping up with the young bucks.

Fortunately, a ray of hope these days is that we, as baby boomers, are not required to "act our age" as much as our parents and grandparents were. Think back to the sixties, and you'll realize that once upon a time, the notion of a 50-year-old rock star would have been inconceivable. Not these days. Mick Jagger, Rod Stewart, Eric Clapton—you name 'em— they're still going strong. Yet suffice it to say that these gents don't live the raucous lifestyle they once had when going on the road. Mick Jagger, for instance, is reputed to work out heftily in order to maintain that requisite endurance for one of his Herculean "farewell" world tours. (He's got another one as I write this.) Adolescence may not ever have to end (in your mind, at least), but you have to work harder to keep whatever version of youthful energy you want to define as your own.

The fact is, sadly enough, that you can't prevent aging. It just happens. The secret is to make this reality as gentle and unobtrusive a process for yourself as possible. I'm a staunch believer in the adage "It's not so much a matter of adding more years to your life as putting more life into your years."

Changes in the Lungs

As in most parts of the body, as you age you're going to notice a certain amount of inevitable decline in the function of your breathing machinery. However, unless you've been a high-level endurance athlete all your life, this change is not so dire as to make you miserable. In fact, if you're an average citizen, you can easily manage to the point of not even noticing those changes.

So what should you expect in terms of lung function? Here's the list, for better or for worse:

- a 25 percent decline in the lungs' vital capacity—that is, the maximum amount of air the lungs can hold.
- a decrease in the ventilation-to-perfusion ratio—the ratio of air to blood in the lungs. This means that the lung tissue ends up getting supplied less efficiently with blood.
- an increase in residual volume—the amount of air left in the lungs after a complete expiration.
- a reduction in the flexibility of the chest wall as the movable ribs calcify. This is called chest wall compliance.
- a decrease in the elastic recoil of the lungs.
- a 50 percent increase in reserve volume between ages 17 and 70.
- an increase in premature airway closure.
- a decrease in amount of alveolar air.
- a decrease in gas transfer.
- a decrease in power of the respiratory muscles.
- a 50 percent decrease in ventilatory response to oxygen/carbon dioxide ratio.

Whew!

In plain English, what this list means is that as you age, your lung tissue becomes less flexible and less able to absorb oxygen. Your lungs don't pump quite as efficiently, hold as much air, or put as much oxygen into your blood. All this is going to happen no matter what you do. How much it affects your life, though, is up to you. No matter how old you are, you can try as best you can to monitor your pulmonary function status, but in later life, guessing pulmonary function becomes harder. Unfortunately, aging lungs can begin to act like the lungs of someone with emphysema. They can become less elastic, less distensible—in other words, less able to stretch.

The so-called small airways—the ones that can become overreactive in asthma or become overly irritable and spasmodic when you least want it—begin to snap closed. The telltale wheezes of asthma are the early closure of these smaller airways.

Along with the so-called ventilation-perfusion mismatch, there is also a loss of muscle power from weaker accessory breathing muscles. That, along with the reduction in lung elasticity, can result in the retention of carbon dioxide, which can contribute to a buildup of lactic acid—the stuff that makes your muscles "burn" when you exercise.

Fortunately, most of the truly bothersome changes to the lungs make their appearance much later in life. Once again, it really does pay to be physically active. For instance, you can lessen calcification of the movable ribs while maintaining their flexibility through exercise and stretching. And an active life can have a beneficial effect on the efficiency of your oxygen consumption.

Then there's the standard caveat—*don't smoke*. Even with nonsmokers, lung capacity drops each year starting anywhere between ages 20 and 35. And airflow, as measured by peak expiratory flow rate and forced expiratory volume (the amount of air you can push out in a second), also declines with age. Smoking only hastens the aging process. Indeed, one of the greatest challenges and potential triumphs for those of us in medical practice can be convincing patients to stop smoking. In every way imaginable, *the health of your lungs demands that you not smoke.*

An ongoing theme I want to stress is that the various parts of your body are interrelated. For example, at the same time lung capacity and function start to decline with age, the rest of your body, especially if it's running poorly, may actually be putting *increased* demands on your lungs. As you age, your fast-twitch muscle fibers (what Michael Johnson and the 200 yard dash are all about) are decreasing. Understandably, there is also a simultaneous decrease in anaerobic muscle enzyme activity. Meanwhile, happily, your slow-twitch fibers, the stuff marathoners are made of, increase with age. But they tend to work efficiently only if you have sufficient oxygen available, and that depends on adequately functioning lungs to deliver the goods.

As we age, we can end up with a body that works less efficiently but demands as much or more lung capacity to accomplish the task. By the time you're passing the 40 mark in that great race of life, even if you had not planned it, you find that you're definitely made for distance, not speed, especially if you can maintain the discipline necessary to maintain fit lung and intercostal muscle tissue. In many ways, there's nothing bad about that.

Another side effect of the big lung change of life and aging is that the respiratory center in the brain that controls breathing can become more sensitive to a drop in oxygen level (called hypoxia) yet tolerate persistently elevated carbon dioxide levels. This is why you may have more trouble sleeping with advancing age. Again, translated into plain English, this means you no longer react to the usual stimuli such as borderline low oxygen or high ambient carbon dioxide levels. You compensate by continuing to take deep breaths or sigh as you sleep. Fortunately, however, for most of us this is more an inconvenience than a serious health problem. Another miracle: You close your eyes, fall asleep, go on automatic pilot, and even wake up the next morning. I've marveled at this process since childhood.

To sum up, your lungs will undergo an inevitable loss of elasticity. Likewise, the muscles of respiration can, if allowed, become as deconditioned as any other muscle in your body. But again, there are steps you can take to minimize these negative effects, steps that I will discuss in later chapters.

Is Arthritis Inevitable ?

Among the most commonly lamented disorders associated with age are "creaking" and painful joints. Most of us have begun to experience at least a little pain after exercise, especially if we haven't stretched properly beforehand, if we haven't exercised for a while, or if we tend to overdo it. To exacerbate the problem, some old athletic injuries can return to try to rob us of physical prowess, our sense of well-being, and even sleep.

There are many causes of joint pain and disability. Some are avoidable—even self-inflicted. Others come to us in spite of our best efforts. Often, we can do something about joint disorders, either through exercise and stretching or with medical treatment. Arthritis—a painful swelling and inflammation of any of the joints in our body—can occur at any age. Disorders of our joints can produce pain, stiffness, swelling, redness, and increased warmth or lead to limited range of motion. Arthritis in one or more of our joints may be due to a systemic (whole body) illness such as one of sever forms of arthritis.

Arthritis can be caused by hemorrhage into a joint, as in hemophilia; by trauma, or from sepsis, due to several not-so-rare bacterial or fungal infections; or by the crystal-induced affliction of gout. Some forms of arthritis are acute and self-limiting, whereas others are chronic. The crucial message is that both the acute and chronic varieties can lead to joint destruction unless properly treated.

There are many ways the inflammation of arthritis can affect your joints. It may hit the small distal (end) joints of your fingers, as in osteoarthritis. More than 40 million Americans (85 percent over age 70) have evidence of osteoarthritis, a chronic form of arthritis that can be easily detected by X ray and exam.

Arthritis may involve the proximal joints of the hand and the covering (synovia) around the wrists, as in rheumatoid arthritis. It may be symmetrical, affecting both sides of the body equally, as in rheumatoid arthritis and osteoarthritis. It may be migratory, as in rheumatic fever, which is usually associated with the signs and symptoms of an acute febrile illness such as Group A strep throat. Rheumatic fever usually affects two or more joints at any one time. Fortunately, rheumatic fever is easily treated and should only be suspected when your throat hurts more than it should, your breath smells fetid, you might be covered with a coalescent (scarlatina form) rash, and you have some funky joint inflammation.

In the earlier decades of life, rheumatoid arthritis affects three times as many women as men, but this equalizes with age, meaning men over 40 are affected with increasing frequency. Rheumatic fever is an insidious illness that starts with fatigue, weakness, joint stiffness, and pain, even before the joints begin to swell. Although 10 to 20 percent of the population who get joint pain and swelling from rheumatic fever can achieve a full recovery, at least 10 percent can go on to a relentless, crippling illness characterized by the destruction of the hands and larger joints due to the spread of inflamed tissue overlying the cartilage. Treatment ranges from aspirin products and steroids to the antimalarials (Chloroquin), gold salts, and even anticancer drugs that delay excessive tissue growth causing the inflammation.

Aging can also bring on an all too common affliction called degenerative joint disease, which is the result of simple wear and tear, with degenerative changes to the cartilage in the joints. If you happen to be an air hammer operator, you could develop this in your elbows or shoulders. Swinging a tennis racquet, throwing a baseball, or double-poling around a cross-country ski course could hasten the disease in the elbows, especially if you're prone to swinging wrong, throwing too hard, or skiing too long.

The knee is a particularly suspect joint. Running, of course, can adversely affect the knees, as do basketball, racquetball, and bicycling. Even walking around a golf course affects the knee. Heck, for all we know, sitting at the breakfast table sipping coffee could adversely affect your knees. In fact, if the knee had been designed by an engineer, he or she would have been fired years ago. Not to make a knee-jerk reaction, the simple moral of the story is to be aware as possible of your body so as not to overstress it.

Another bread-and-butter yet infuriating variety of joint disease is carpal tunnel syndrome, an overuse process that adversely affects the covering of your wrist tendons. Resulting pain stems from compression of the median nerve to your hand as it travels through an increasingly unyielding carpal tunnel with the other nerves and tendon bundles of the wrist. Characteristically, those who suffer from this painful, frequently nocturnal malady have a numbness or burning sensation from the palm into the thumb, index, and middle fingers. Those who repetitively flex or extend their wrists are most susceptible. Anti-inflammatory drugs or a wrist support (a cock-up splint) will sometimes help avoid or at least delay surgical decompression of this tunnel. Occasionally, a steroid shot under the wrist covering (the flexor retinaculum) can help avoid or at least delay sometimes inevitable surgery.

Most men ought to know about Reiter's syndrome, a condition characterized by a triad of arthritis, conjunctivitis, and urethritis. Fortunately, it is less common if you're over 40. It is, in point of fact, an affliction of young studs. Ten percent of cases can be caused by a partner's vaginal infection, and 90 percent by food poisoning. Symptoms may occur a few days to four weeks after sex. Fortunately, this form of arthritis may respond well to relatively safe anti-inflammatory drugs such as Indocin or other nonsteroidals such as ibuprofen (Advil). The attendant and somewhat nerve-wracking urethritis ("the drip") can be treated successfully with tetracycline, which works well for almost any nonspecific urethral infection (NSU).

Infection is nothing to mess around with, especially when it involves one of your joints. Septic arthritis, specifically, is a medical emergency your doctor must recognize and treat immediately to avoid permanent damage to one of your joints. Your doctor should remove fluid from the infected joint quickly, analyze it, have the fluid cultured, and, if necessary, begin antibiotic treatment posthaste. Last, when an infection in a vital joint just isn't improving, open surgical drainage may be necessary. That's the time to call in the surgeon.

Gout goes back to Hippocrates, the legendary father of medicine, 2,500 years before our much-maligned Pickwickian gourmand ever began stuffing his face with sweetbreads only to grab an exquisitely painful big toe shortly thereafter. Gout is caused by the buildup of uric acid crystals, especially in the first joint of the toe. It is primarily a disease of adult men, uncommon before the third decade, but with a peak incidence in the fifth decade. Gout tends to run a painful course caused by elevation of uric acid, the product of purine or DNA breakdown, culminating in painful, gouty arthritis. Between attacks, gout crystals tend to deposit painlessly in the joints.

A high uric acid level in the blood can also cause indescribably painful kidney stones. Some women have compared these minuscule monsters to labor pains. Medically, there is an association between a high uric acid level with gout, obesity, hypertension, diabetes, and abnormal lipids, cholesterol, and triglyceride.

There is no easy answer to joint pain. What's good for one type of disorder may only make another one worse. For example, the physical activity that helps the arthritis victim maintain motion in the affected joints can only make the pain of degenerative joint disease worse.

If you experience joint pain, don't get too worked up unnecessarily. The afflictions I mentioned aren't necessarily as dire as you think. A case of garden-variety arthritis, for example, can be treated with a medication as simple as aspirin. Obviously, early diagnosis and intervention can make all the difference between temporary, intermittent joint pain and painful, ultimately dysfunctional joint destruction. Recognizing the problem, seeking medical consultation, and pursuing the most logical solution is the commonsense approach.

Low Back Pain

According to neurosurgeon and low back pain specialist Dr. Chuck Burton of the Minneapolis Institute for Low Back Care, the normal back typically becomes dysfunctional by the time we reach the age of 50 to 60. This could seem like some mighty depressing information. However, I'm 52, and I do everything almost without a suggestion of back pain.

Much of what goes wrong, says Burton, has a great deal to do with the hostile environment of our planet—the high gravitational force of Mother Earth (on our back), compounded by such correctable factors as a sedentary lifestyle, poor nutrition, plus stress and a boatload of bad habits, such as smoking and drinking too much. For many of us, unfortunately, this is a lot of what life can be all about. Mine was.

In only 2 percent of acute back problems is an initial specific diagnosis ever actually made. Eighty percent of people who have acute back pain manage to get better without any medical help. However, the cost while you are waiting for that to happen spontaneously is $6,000 or so, what with lost work, medications, and other bills. So the goal is to screen out all those with a specific diagnosis, treating all the rest with an effective conservative back program. More on the specifics about that in a moment.

There are several theories about what causes our lower backs to give us such trouble.

Theory 1—Too Much Stress Can Do It

It is difficult to document, but easy to believe, that there are stressors or psychological events that build up in your life until your body says, "Help! I've got to stop, I'm on overload!" Perhaps it is a collection of overwhelming events in your life that can precipitate back pain. On a subconscious level, perhaps it is far easier to accept disabling back pain than the reality of the stressors possibly responsible.

Theory 2—A Poor Physical State of Health

Poor physical health can also make you an easy setup for an attack of back pain. There are two possible reasons for this. First, as you age, you may not maintain abdominal musculature in the kind of shape necessary to complement those workhorses, the deep paravertebral muscles of the back, nestled deep and along your posterior spine. The reality is that many of us are just not willing to take the little extra time necessary to either stretch or strengthen our backs. Practically every comparative study shows as well that worksite educational programs decrease absenteeism and perceived pain in workers unlucky enough to get injured. Nurturing your back often ends up taking a backseat to the everyday tasks of daily living: endlessly driving the kids and the long list of tasks required of husbands and fathers. Sometimes, if you need motivation, simply a session with a physical therapist, personal trainer, or chiropractor can help you recover faster while teaching you tricks to building your extensor muscles as well as stronger abs.

By the time you are 50, says Burton, your spine has already begun to metamorphose, so that you could be vulnerable to injury due to friable intervertebral discs, especially if you have battered your body lifting wrong or falling. If you are in this category, you may already have built plenty of little calcified outcroppings jutting out from your vertebrae, just waiting to pinch unsuspecting nerves emerging from your spinal cord on their mission to innervate your hamstrings, foot flexors, calves, or toes. The sciatic notch, where those nerves pass through on their journey south to your thigh or leg, can suddenly become a beacon of pain if aggravated.

So who can help you the most? Lest we physicians become self-righteous, all types of health providers are similar in terms of times to functional recovery. What is most interesting, however, is the cost of health care services. Outpatient charges were highest for chiropractors and orthopedists and lowest for HMO and primary-care providers.

Theory 3—The "Live Life Dangerously Factor"

This can often be part of "counterphobic" behavior of midlife. We're talking hang gliding, bungee jumping (with or without a bungee), dangerous liaisons (right place, right time, wrong woman concept), or taking up car racing or ski jumping at age 40. But there is often a renewed reluctance to believe we are mortal similar to those wild and crazy days of late adolescence and shortly thereafter.

Many of us can end up enjoying the sport of our choice—golf, tennis (so-called unidirectional sports), jogging, waterskiing—in ways that could end up producing low back pain. Certain sports, such as golf or tennis, include a notorious twisting motion. Especially if done with the enthusiasm of a teenager and the body of a 40 year old, this new avocation could pull, rip, or severely strain many of those structural small muscles, tendons, ligaments, or bones in your low back.

Still others of those repetitively jarring or grinding passions, such as jogging, high-impact aerobics, and even mogul jumping, can wear down not only your bones but also your intervertebral discs, those cushions between vertebrae so structurally vital that show such horrendous consequences if they become pissed off. By the luck of the wrong draw, you could end up either temporarily or permanently disabled.

A siege of severe low-back pain can start innocently, just from bending, swinging, lifting, carrying, jumping, sneezing, or intercourse. Just sitting in an airplane seat may be all that some people—and especially tall ones—need. It may often be difficult, if not impossible, for you to sort out just what is wrong with you other than the reality that your back hurts like hell, you can't move, and you can hardly find a comfortable position. Like a wounded animal, you soon discover that lying very still in the fetal position, with your legs curled up against your chest, may be the only possible way you will ever survive. Have someone place pillows under your knees to relieve some of the stretch on your sciatic nerve and some of that painful torque on the deep muscles in your back.

If you end up in the emergency room, your doctor there will immediately assess just how severe your pain really is and, if necessary, try to relieve the pain with a shot of any of a number of preparations that can make your life temporarily livable again (assuming you are not allergic to any of them): They can include Toradol, Demerol, morphine, or a combination of the above.

Such an aggressive initial approach to treating acute and even intolerable back pain can make your doctor's subsequent neurological examination possible. The trauma to the specific part of your back can show up in the body part the affected nerve supplies. Your clinician will check your knee reflexes to determine if your third or fourth lumbar nerves are injured. The fifth lumbar nerve can be checked by seeing how your big toe lifts upward. Finally, ankle jerks help test for an injury of your first sacral nerve roots. Wow, we've practically got you halfway through medical school already. All this sounds very technical, but when you are really hurting, there can be a lot of overlap of symptoms or findings, so it is important from the outset to relieve your pain even if it is transitory.

Your physician can learn a great deal by lifting your lower leg while your thigh is flexed up toward your chest. This test is called Lesegue's Sign, named after the Frenchman who first discovered another way of torturing you. This maneuver stretches the third lumbar nerve root as it meanders out through your sciatic notch. It is an easy diagnostic test your doc can do while you are lying flat on your back, which is usually your position of choice anyway and the extent of movement you'll want to undergo.

In this age of legalistic medicine, your physician will most likely order front and side views of your lumbar spine. These X rays are low on the yield side both in specificity and sensitivity. Lumbar spine films are one way of early on detecting forward slippage (spondylolisthesis) of one of your lumbar vertebrae over another or an arch defect (fracture) posteriorly without actual slippage (spondylolysis). Your physician can also see "lipping"—that is, growths around individual vertebrae due to osteoarthritis or narrowing of your intervertebral disc spaces from this or an earlier degenerative process or injury.

In the majority of cases, you may have an abnormal X ray or, at worst, an X ray that shows chronic degenerative changes of the spine from aging. The best treatment is still usually conservative: positioning yourself comfortably with your legs flexed over some pillows and taking a nonsteroidal anti-inflammatory potion such as ibuprofen in doses of 600 or 800 milligrams, four or three times a day, respectively, that is, if your stomach can tolerate it.

You may require other medications such as muscle relaxants to reduce swelling and spasm. Your physician may choose any of several other stronger options, including some major pain pills such as Tylenol with codeine for when the pain really gets bad, as it often does at night. There are times when these medicines can really make the difference. Remember to reinforce *pain-free* intervals rather than the *pain-full* moments. Put simply, take your pain medications regularly, and not just when you hurt during one of these sieges.

During your first week with a pulled back, your physician may choose to emphasize pain relief, rest, and comfort (survival) care. By the second week, he or she may send you to physical therapy for hot packs, massage, electrical stimulation, and ultrasound. The touch and caring of a physical therapist or massage therapist can do amazing things toward speeding your healing process, especially as therapy relaxes the spasm going throughout your body without any sense or direction. Now is the time to have whoever is giving you care to attack the spasm in the extensor muscles of your back by stretching them: using contrast therapy (ice and heat), giving you low-voltage electrical stimulation, or employing low-weight, high-repetition resistance exercises. As one doctor notes, "emphasize strengthening the extensors to offset the world we live in putting us in flexion most of the day." Seeing a chiropractor is often very helpful.

Now might be the time to return to theory 1 and to think about the stressors in your life and healthy ways for relieving them. Also consider beginning a home back-strengthening program with weight loss—if necessary—to further minimize degenerative changes perhaps responsible for this whole vicious cycle in the first place. Consider, too, that the weakest link in the back structure may be your abdominal muscles. These may have gone to pot (literally) since you last needed them for high school football. Oh, those sixties.

Once your acute back pain subsides, throwing in different types of tummy crunches once or twice a day to strengthen your jelly belly could do a lot toward rebuilding your back in a healthy body, and a happy spirit.

Down With Fat Old Men (Why We Really Gain Weight)

If we're really honest with ourselves, we'll admit that aside from nagging thoughts about a sudden or painful death, the aspect of aging that concerns many of us the most is that we simply don't look like ourselves anymore. Somehow, having our significant others tweak us fondly on one of our chins and exclaim, "There's more of you to love," may not always be entirely comforting. Although a certain amount of weight gain invariably occurs with aging, you are responsible for determining the ceiling.

Why does everything have to head south as we age? Although muscles do weaken and atrophy with age, they will still respond very favorably by strengthening and regaining strength with physical conditioning (more about that in chapter 6). As we age, there is an inevitable decline in the amount of muscle mass as it is replaced by adipose tissue (fat). That's why simply maintaining your weight into middle age may not be as impressive an accomplishment as it may seem. The fat on board weighs less, leaving the unthinkable possibility that a once fit, now overweight man could get fat and actually lose weight. This is why I am especially disturbed by actuarial tables that so routinely allow for weight gain with age—they underestimate our actual weight gain. I prefer Body Mass Index (BMI), which is a ratio of body weight to height.

The result of this endorsement of obesity by insurance companies is that the older American becomes not only hopelessly less fit, but fatter—yet still manages to qualify as acceptable to the insurance company. What a deal. But why does this happen in the first place? Is the replacement of all that nice muscle with fat an inevitable and natural process that we can do nothing about?

Not necessarily. As we age, our lifestyles become imperceptibly more sedentary. This causes our metabolisms to slow, causing our dinners to end up somewhere around our waists. Don't forget that the average American wouldn't run for a bus. I read recently that the famous Rhodes Scholar and Knicks player-turned-Senator couldn't run 3 miles. Pity.

But it's not all our fault. When muscle tone becomes harder to maintain, exercising seems more difficult, and we avoid it. Then, too, there's the lifestyle that our careers and families enforce on us. We sit at work; we sit taking our kids here or there. Just remember, if your family loves you, they will let you have time to exercise. And if your bosses care about their health insurance rates, they will, too.

John Bland, MD, emeritus professor of rheumatology at the University of Vermont, sounds an optimistic note when he promises that people over 40 have to do fewer strengthening exercises to achieve the same effect as their younger counterparts. It takes less effort, says Bland, to gain in fitness with conditioning as we get older. Also, he says with glee, oldsters decondition slower than younger peers.

So rather than the few weeks an idle Olympian will take to deteriorate into a deconditioned state, the older master ski racer, for instance, may hang in there for months, bless his soul.

Here is also one place where men have the advantage over women. It takes relatively small amounts of exercise or just an improved diet for most men to shed the pounds. On the other hand, studies show that at midlife women must both adhere to a strict low-fat diet and engage in frequent high-intensity aerobic exercise to have the same effect. Who said life was fair?

Osteo What? Do Your Bones Really Change?

Here's another bit of good news: Although bone mass declines progressively after your fourth decade, positive efforts such as exercise can slow or, in some cases, even reverse the process. Though this is reputed to be more of a problem for women, osteoporosis and loss of bone mass do afflict men as well, especially those who are sedentary. And lest we fantasize that we are still 18, a word of caution: Demineralization may make it easier to break bones. Take precautions, use good judgment, and maybe think twice before bungee jumping.

Only His Hairdresser Knows for Sure (Or: Where Does Your Hair Really Go After Forty?)

Another of the real bêtes noires for most men is hair loss. It is little comfort that endocrinologists assure us the guy with the most testosterone surging through his body is the one who balds fastest—so-called android alopecia (male hormone baldness).

We continue to live in a very youth-oriented society, which explains why there is so great a sale of toupees or hair weaves, not to mention what sounds like plenty expensive and moderately uncomfortable hair transplants from the hidden areas on the back of the scalp to other places most in need.

Even if you're not losing your hair, that's not to say you're out of the tonsorial woods. What hair you keep, be it most of it or little of it, will probably turn white.

Equality ends there, however. Some of you will turn gray in your thirties; others will hang in with plenty of youthful pigment until much later. Why does hair turn gray at different stages of life for everyone? Loss of pigment in your hair, meaning turning gray, is caused by a decrease in active melanocytes (responsible for color pigmentation) in your hair bulbs. Whether it happens early or late is mere luck of the draw. When did your dad, granddad, or uncle turn gray? That can give you a clue what your fate will be.

S-E-X

Although sex just ain't the same as we age, there may be easily reversible physical reasons for the shortfall. Urologists tell us that half of impotent men—men who can't achieve or maintain an erection adequate for vaginal penetration—could have a physical reason for what need not be their personal hell. It is unfortunate that so many of us judge our manliness by either the hardness or perceived length of our penises. This gestalt may explain advertisements for having your penis enlarged or why it makes sense to have a surgeon surgically implant a plastic dowel or inflatable pouch into the shaft of your penis.

"Impotence, however, is not 'normal' or 'healthy.' Physically active men.... with an available partner can enjoy sexual intimacy and intercourse well into old age," says physician Neil H. Baum of New Orleans in *Geriatric Medicine News and Reports*. Now this is sounding optimistic.

Our understanding about sexual function in men is that a major factor for the likelihood our machinery will function properly has most to do with regular use over the years. I do have a little bit of bad news, gentlemen, those who thought I was going to offer the fountain of youth for erections. Alas, there is a geometric, steady, and inexorable increase in erectile dysfunction with age—that is, 10 percent by age 50, 30 percent by age 60, 60 percent by age 70, and over 90 percent in all men over 80, according to Baum. How old were Charlie Chaplin, Cary Grant, and Tony Randall when they had their first occurrence of impotence—if at all?

At our tender age, 40, impotence can reliably be taken as a sign of some problem or other, usually a physical one. A fairly rapid onset of sexual dysfunction should alert men to the early signs of a vascular or neurological disease. Impotence can even be an early predictor of coronary artery disease.

Baum describes the normal physiologic changes associated with erection and aging:

1. It takes longer amounts of genital stimulation to get aroused.
2. The refractory period—time from ejaculation to the next erection—takes longer. (We're not necessarily getting better, but we're taking longer, which in some cases has a lot to say favorably compared with the hundredths of a second frenzy of our youth.)

3. There is a decrease in force of ejaculation. (Who cares? An orgasm is an orgasm, is an orgasm.)
4. There is a decrease in the volume of ejaculation.
5. There is more rapid detumescense after ejaculation. (Again, so what.)
6. There is a decreased need to have an ejaculation or orgasm with every coital experience. "Oh, so unselfish."

Say you're one of those guys who is starting to have problems. You may have a variety of reactions, but unfortunately, denial may be pretty high on the list. That's too bad because your problem is very likely to be physical and curable. So you have to decide if you want to get help.

If the answer is yes, then a detailed sexual history can be very helpful. It is frequently helpful to have your partner there as someone asks these questions. A drug history that includes finding out if you consume too much alcohol, tobacco, and illicit, over-the-counter, or prescription drugs is crucial. It is not unusual for one or more of these to be a principal offender. The good news here is if that's the case, the problem can be easily correctable just by stopping it.

Watch your blood pressure and, if you're on certain antihypertensive medications as simple as a diuretic, consult your physician and consider stopping it. A physical examination should always include a thorough genito-urinary examination. This means the doctor examines all of you, including doing a rectal to feel your prostate (especially if you are over 40). You should also be checked for signs of diabetes, kidney function, or low testosterone. Should your doctor confirm that your problem is indeed physical, then you will likely be referred to a urologist (a physician who specializes in the genitourinary tract) for further evaluation.

The midlife experience may bring depression, another bugaboo that can affect a man's sexual function (see the section on depression in the next chapter). Just getting a patient off certain medications and replacing them with one of the newer, less problematic ones can eradicate this frightening development in any man's forties. A big part of a cure can be as simple as acceptance both for the victim and for his partner.

Once you and your physician eliminate any reversible cause of our impotence, oral medications (such as Yohimbine and Viagra), hopefully relatively painless injections into your bulbar cavernosus underneath your penis, and even surgical implants are available to combat erection difficulties.

Viagra has received big-time press since its debut. But what is this stuff that makes impotent men get up on their hind quarters and howl like a wolf for a prescription?

Viagra (sildenafil citrate) does not directly cause penile erections. Instead, it affects a man's response to sexual stimulation. The drug enhances the effects of nitric oxide, a chemical normally released by the body in response to sexual stimulation. Nitric oxide relaxes the smooth muscles and widens the blood vessels in the penis, increasing blood flow and enabling an erection to occur.

Viagra pills come in 25-, 50-, and 100-milligram doses. The maximum dosing frequency is once per day. For most men, the recommended dose for Viagra is 50 mg taken, as needed, approximately 1 hour before sexual activity. If you are not sexually stimulated, nothing will happen. But at $10 a pill, that can be costly in more ways than one.

While Viagra is unquestionably more desirable to use than surgical implants or medications that must be injected, there are potential health hazards and side effects associated with this new manna, including headaches, flushing, indigestion, and visual disturbances that are usually mild. You should not take Viagra if you take drugs known as nitrates, in any form, at any time. One of the most commonly used nitrates is nitro-glycerin, which is frequently prescribed for angina (chest pain due to heart disease). Nitrates can lower blood pressure to unsafe levels if used with Viagra. There are some other medications (Tagamet, erythromycin, and ketoconazole) that, taken simultaneously, could spell trouble by delaying breakdown and increasing plasma concentrations.

All in all, though, for any man unable to produce an erection on demand, Viagra offers some potential (albeit expensive) help. The biggest kahuna of all medical journals, *The New England Journal of Medicine,* in a recent commentary using the International Index of Erectile Function, found that men did better in the erection arena using Viagra than those who didn't.

If you do experience erection difficulties, your regular physician or a urologist can go into details during a consultation about what will work for you. No matter what, keep in mind that there are many ways to thread a needle. Some are actually a lot of fun.

SUGGESTED READINGS

Arnot, Bob. *Dr. Bob Arnot's Guide to Turning Back the Clock.* Little Brown, 1995. 403 pp.

Bland, John H., *Live Long, Die Fast: Playing the Aging Game to Win.* Fairview Press, 1997. 240 pp.

Long, James W. *The Guide to Chronic Illness.* Harper Perennial, 1997. 625 pp.

The Medical Advisor: The Complete Guide to Alternative and Conventional Treatments. Time-Life, 1997. 1,152 pp.

Rippe, James M. *Fit Over 40.* Quill, 1996. 348 pp.

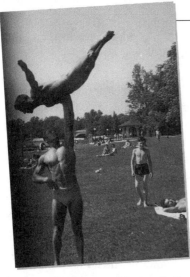

Norm Oakvik

His advice: Continue sports and working out

Norm Oakvik is about the only septuagenarian I know who manages to fall off his bike when out for the last ride of the season. The bad news is that he falls off. The good news is that Norm doesn't break anything. He attributes this stroke of luck to strong muscles. "I could have broken my hip," he says. "All my bones are getting brittle. Everyone in my family has had osteoporosis—my mother, my grandmother." Nevertheless, there are a lot of sprained muscles, which puts him on crutches for a while.

Norm grew up in Minnesota as one of several children of Norwegian-born parents, his father a carpenter from Mosjen, a town way up near the Arctic Circle, and his mother a nurse from the outskirts of Oslo. His father took Norm out to a ski jump in a Minneapolis park, introducing him to a sport at which he would later excel. In fact, he became so enamored with jumping that it was not unusual for him to walk the four miles to the park carrying his skis. When he wasn't jumping, he pursued gymnastics and wrestling, winning the AAU weight lifting championship in the late forties and early fifties. Norm loved to hit the beach and impress the first with human pyramids and other gymnastic feats. (See the photo above.)

As he grew older, Norm began to excel in cross-country skiing as well, taking the North American Championships in Ishpeming in 1954, and the Nordic Combined Championships (cross-country and jumping) in 1955. In the 1960s, he added bicycling to his competitive sports, competing in 60- and 100-mile races. Moving into the late 1970s and early 1980s, Norm continued to excel in America's own cross-country skiing North American Birkebeiner, racing six times and winning his age class twice. In 1996, at age 73, he traveled to Europe to ski the famous 58-kilometer Norwegian Birkebeiner. "I just toured it," he comments with his usual humility, but his time was an impressive 5 1/2 hours. This is all from a guy who weighed 110 pounds at the end of high school and at his best 135 when lifting weights.

Yet Norm has had his down time, too. He broke his ankle once ski jumping and his wrist on another occasion while falling off a scaffold as a sheet metal worker. "I was way up and came down head first," he says.

"I'm just lucky I'm alive." Though a hip replacement five years ago ended his competitive career, it hasn't stopped him from getting back on his cross-country skis or mounting his all-terrain bike.

Norm strongly advocates the benefits of weight lifting for older athletes, knowing full well that loss of muscle mass is a consequence of growing older. As for diet, he says, "I eat plenty of protein and carbohydrates in the form of breads and cereals, including oatmeal almost every morning. I eat well. But even if I eat fattening foods, I don't gain weight." Norm is fortunate on this score, but no doubt part of the reason is his active lifestyle.

"So what's my advice for anyone over 40?" He saves me the trouble of asking. "Continue sports and working out. Remember to maintain good muscle tone using weights. Of course, I'm nuts about cross-country skiing. In those times of inactivity and slowing down, it's so important to keep up activity, to keep your muscles in good shape. Most people my age are decrepit from a sedentary lifestyle. Exercise and keeping in shape keeps your mind sharp as well."

At a diminutive 124 pounds, Norm Oakvik still skis with power and grace. That is, when he's not on crutches from a bicycling mishap. He smiles as I chide him that he has to work on his road sports. We both know that he'll be back on his skis with the first big snow of the season.

■ *Chapter 3*

What to Expect
From Your Nerves

In the name of Hippocrates, doctors have invented the most exquisite
form of torture ever known to man: survival.

Luis Bunuel, Spanish filmmaker, *My Last Sigh*

Another slow change that is variable from one man to another in midlife is a
"desensitizing" of your nervous system. Let's call it a slowly changing
process, but there are a few nagging chronic—as well as a couple of more
acute—issues that could begin to trouble you.

One is simply a slower reaction time. In most cases, we may not even
notice it. In the days of the woolly mammoth, your edge could make a big
difference at mealtimes whether you were the diner or the dinner.

Your nerves are the electrical wiring to your entire body, and there are a
number of related issues involving your nerves that become more important to you as you pass 40. The aging of the nervous system figures critically
in illnesses that become more prevalent with age. And there are a number
of such ailments affecting nerves that can become quite devastating.

When or If Your Nerves Go "Boing"
Hereditary Disorders
It is important to probe into your lineage. Although Huntington's disease,
for instance, characterized by progressive, irregular, random movements
and dementia, occurs in adulthood, the causes are very much hereditary.
Diseases like this can be a deeply hidden secret lurking in your family tree
that appears surreptitiously owing to late onset, denial, errors due to
incorrect paternity, or variable expression (of these traits).

A fairly simple view of hereditary diseases deals with the types of genes,
dominant or recessive, that are inherited from parents. Dominant characteristics can be inherited from one parent, but recessive characteristics
must come from both parents. Dominant diseases, therefore, show strong
generation-to-generation patterns, whereas recessive ones can skip one or
more generation or disappear entirely.

Nonhereditary Disorders

In people afflicted with the neuropathies (debilitating conditions involving larger nerves of the body), 50 percent of the time a thorough medical examination will reveal diabetes mellitus, alcohol abuse, chronic kidney disease, a nutritional deficiency, the presence of a toxic drug, cancer, or a connective tissue disease. Forty percent of the remainder end up with a genetically determined neuropathy.

Seizures

Seizures are what happen when your brain neurons suddenly go crazy. Though sudden and frightening, most episodes are brief. Fortunately, seizures aren't something that most of us have to worry about, but that doesn't mean we should forget about them altogether. They can occur for the first time in adults over 40. Classic tonic-clonic (gran mal) seizures, during which individuals bite their tongues involuntarily, wet their pants, or whack their heads badly enough to require stitches, can occur in persons of every age.

The rule of thumb is that any individual who shows up in the emergency room with a bona fide seizure deserves a complete neurological workup: an EEG, a CAT scan or a magnetic resonance imaging study (MRI), or even the new positive emission tomography (PET), and a spinal tap to rule out an intracranial bleed, an infection, or cancer. Certain types of seizures can result from an infectious process such as encephalitis, or a metabolic problem such as low blood sugar, lack of oxygen, or even alcohol withdrawal. There are also partial seizures (petit mal) from metabolic abnormalities, or partial complex seizures (psychomotor temporal lobe seizures) that can show very different symptoms such as memory loss, amnesia, or momentary lapses in alertness.

There are many causes of seizures, so don't assume anything. Get it checked out immediately. Running across someone writhing in the street from a full-blown gran mal seizure is enough of a lesson for understanding the severity of seizures. They are unique, often enigmatic, and frightfully dangerous due to such self-inflicted injuries as fractures, concussions, aspiration of food or teeth, or even suffocation.

Parkinson's Disease

Parkinson's disease most often hits in later life but can sneak up during midlife. For example, Muhammad Ali developed this disease at a relatively early age, perhaps due to too many blows to the head. Parkinson's symptoms include a blank, masklike facial expression, a stooped posture, unusually slow movements, tremors at rest, shuffling, and a so-called festinating (quick step) gait—victims appear as though they're walking fast while bent over into a gale wind.

Alzheimer's Disease

Dementias such as Alzheimer's are also more common in later life, but they too can appear at any age. However, take heart: The risks are nothing like the inevitability that you'd suspect from many of the sensational reports on the evening news. This disorder is the cause of 60 percent of all dementias, and almost 25 percent of people over 85 could develop Alzheimer's. As we've already suggested, many of the mental afflictions of aging have other causes. Plenty of patients with morbid depression, for example, have tripped up experts because what they really have is a condition called pseudodementia. It can masquerade as dementia but actually has a more emotional, even treatable, cause.

Dementias have other organic causes, though, such as drug intoxication, hypothyroidism, chronic meningitis, even syphilitic encephalitis, and B_{12}, foliate, or thiamine deficiencies.

Stroke

When a vessel in the brain hemorrhages and blood goes smashing about where it doesn't belong, the result can be irreparable damage to brain tissue. Increased pressure on the brain can have profound effects on the health of the entire nervous system, the brain itself, or, more significantly, actual deadly pressure on the brain stem.

When it comes to the broad and important category of cerebrovascular diseases, the U.S. government's Framingham study, which has tracked more than 5,000 adult residents of Framingham, Massachusetts, since the late 1940s, found hypertension, either systolic or diastolic, to be the most important risk factor producing strokes. Because African-American males demonstrate the highest incidence of essential hypertension (of unknown cause, yet treatable), it should come as no surprise that this same group has the highest incidence of strokes.

Other risk factors that the aging male can eliminate by an occasional visit to the doctor include diabetes, a high cholesterol and triglyceride, or cigarette smoking. The incidence of strokes has declined largely owing to the more vigorous preventive approaches being taken. This may well represent one of the areas where epidemiology and hands-on medicine have worked successfully together to treat disease.

The initial approach to anyone unfortunate enough to have developed a stroke is supportive care. This is because at first there is a great deal of swelling or edema, which can accentuate the severity of the usual findings from a stroke. At its worst, the edema can affect the respiratory center and compromise usually automatic or involuntary breathing.

During this time, steroids and mannitol, a large-molecule sugar, can be given to shrink swelling. During the acute phase of the stroke, there should be careful attention to the breakdown of skin (decubiti), which can develop over mere hours; the prevention of urinary retention; and the psychological needs of the impaired patient. If the stroke involves Broca's speech area on the left side of the brain, the stroke victim usually has an expressive aphasia (unable to express oneself verbally) in addition to a possibly complete flaccid paralysis of the opposite side of the body.

I learned recently with sadness that the director of my own medicine residency program in the late seventies had gotten zapped by a stroke. Keep in mind that numerically, however, blacks, who top the statistics for so-called malignant hypertension, with a diastolic number above 120 and the systolic number above 200, get strokes, whereas whites like my training director usually get heart attacks with their attendant risk factors.

Last I heard, this same individual (who had often made my life miserable as a lowly medical resident) has not improved much. However, a luckier few often experience a watershed phenomenon in which adjacent brain tissue compensates for the area injured by loss of blood supply. Alternatively, stroke victims can experience an internal bleed flooding the live brain with blood and inflammatory fluid.

Unfortunately, a severe headache, one that awakens you out of a peaceful sleep and persists despite your taking mega doses of aspirin, Advil, or Tylenol, could make you suspicious, but not necessarily paranoid, of an intracranial event.

One of my fellow residents had crescendo headache and could literally feel the explosion of blood beginning to blow up his brain. Because he knew that this represented a ruptured cerebral aneurysm and a subsequent hemorrhagic stroke, he called 911 in enough time for a neurosurgeon to "crack" his head to "clip" the bleeder. He would never, however, return to his previous level of practice as a hematologist and subsequently became a pathologist.

There are the plenty who will have a stroke and return to very near their earlier level. The changes may be very subtle: a dragging foot or an arm and hand pulled up and barely functional from contractures. They may have a persistent facial droop, not altogether unlike what one sees in someone with a Bell's (a peripheral seventh cranial nerve) palsy. Classically, someone with a typical central stroke will deflect the movement of their tongue to the side of the stroke.

The name of the game for my training director and my hematologist-turned-pathologist is rehabilitation, rehabilitation, and more rehabilitation. The experts will do what they can with speech therapy, attempts —often not a little painful—at walking, increasing range of motion, and balance.

Contractures would rather not be straightened out. This is where the physical therapist must combine the intensity of an Attila with the gentleness of your mother. Prevention is key. If you have bad hypertension, get it treated. If your father or grandfather has had an arteriovenous malformation (AVM), go get a head MRI; it's the best for soft lesions in the brain.

The Eyes Have It

Or do they? Okay, so your eye problems aren't figments of your imagination. Middle age—that is, turning 40-something—appears to be the critical age for a lot of light-to-moderate nastiness having to do with your eyes. The most noticeable change as we age is in our visual acuity, especially close up, or "near vision." It seems that our arms have become too short. Then, too, as we get older, night driving becomes more difficult because we become hypersensitive to glare. There are other potential problems, but these are the most common.

The dimensions of vision most commonly affected by age are the following:

- visual processing speed (reading speed)
- light sensitivity (the ability to see in twilight or dark)
- dynamic vision (like reading scrolling TV credits)
- near vision (for small print)
- visual search (like locating a sign)

Let's get down to cases. According to Timothy Diegel, MD, clinical associate professor of ophthalmology at the University of Minnesota, "Turning 40 is a time of accommodative weakness." In other words, you experience decreased eye (visual) function but usually adapt to it effectively so that you may not even notice it.

This means many things, from a vision perspective. As we age, for example, the cornea begins to flatten, accentuating any earlier astigmatism. Our lenses, devoid of their own blood supply, are especially sensitive already to any form of insult—traumatic, toxic, or degenerative—and may develop dullness or actual visual disability. With age, we all lose the ability to increase the thickness or curvature of the lens in order to focus on near objects. Tell me about it. You know something's seriously wrong when you have to ask your dinner partner on the other side of the table to hold your menu so that you can read it.

Another hazard of aging is dry eyes. When you're tired or have been exposed to cold air, wind, toxic fumes, or rain, contacts can become unpleasant or impossible to wear. Individuals spend their entire workday within high-rise offices cursed with low humidity and windows that won't open. Humidifiers, of course, are now verboten because of code restrictions. They have been known to cause other inconveniences such as a sometimes fatal pneumonia called Legionnaire's disease. The books say that the average humidity in the Sahara Desert is somewhere in the neighborhood of 37 percent. In the average office building in the wintertime, it's more like 20 percent. Either way, you have to choose between perpetually dry eyes or risk a humidifier and a big-time fine.

Artificial tears or thick rewetting drops are a preventive, if not simplistic, answer to keratoconjunctivitis sicca (dry eyes). If you are going to spend an extended amount of time outdoors, load up on these thick moisteners.

Ever heard of "floaters?" These are vitreous particles, shaped like dots, lines, and even cobwebs, that can make the sun's rays painful to the eyes. In the least, they are distracting, but they can lead to more serious problems. Such possibilities include a retinal detachment, or worse yet, vitreal hemorrhage. If someone has floaters that are in fact annoying, a retinal vitreous surgeon has techniques for removing them by inserting needles (painlessly), aspirating the floaters out, and then replacing the fluid with a balanced salt solution.

Eyelids, too, can literally begin to turn on you in midlife. Eyelids that begin to turn in (entropian) or out (ectropian) may produce excessive tearing or painful redness. Because the eyelids are a perfect barrier catching the sun's rays first, they are also a perfect setup for basal cell carcinoma (that is what a raised, reddening, pearly bump on the eyelid ends up being 90 percent of the time, especially if you are fair-skinned and blue-eyed). The cure for most of these problems of the lids can be straightforward: excision. Fortunately, these are annoying enough that most people don't wait too long before getting them checked out.

Protect your eyes. There are plenty of state-of-the-art breakproof (polycarbonate) lenses and breakaway frames that will not become a part of your permanent bone structure in a face plant. They can also prevent a lacerated eyeball from a ski pole tip or a swinging branch.

Some eye problems, such as near visual acuity trouble, can easily be overcome by getting reading glasses or bifocals. The others you may just have to get used to, just as you have of all those wrinkles you see in the mirror every morning.

Hearing: Is It Getting Worse, or Are You Just Not Listening?

Hearing impairment with age can be normally mild or moderate in severity, yet it tends to be a widespread problem. Such problems begin to show up in midlife. These difficulties have a number of causes and can have various effects. In some cases, as in losses in ability to hear high-pitched sound, the causes are self-inflicted, stemming from having sampled too many rock concerts. Other problems are hereditary in nature. Still others are due to normal changes associated with aging that affect all of us differently.

Background Noise

As we age, we lose the ability to tune out background noises. Consequently, we frequently have greater difficulty hearing in noisy settings. This would affect your ability to hear a friend trying to get your attention across a crowded room. This is a difficult problem to overcome. Hearing aids tend to amplify sound indiscriminately, leaving up to you the problem of separating those sounds you want to hear from those you don't. You can only hope that your particular case is mild and uncomplicated by other hearing problems.

High-Pitch Hearing Loss

There are plenty of reasons why anyone who has spent time around high-pitched noises ends up testing positive for high-frequency hearing loss. Call it "rock 'n roller's ear." Individuals working around foundries, boiler making, or loud noises such as gunfire may also flunk hearing tests for high-pitched frequencies. Such problems, fortunately, may be treatable with a myriad of types of hearing aids or, as a last resort, surgery. Researchers even have developed an implantable synthetic cochlea (the balance center of the ear) already.

More important, high-pitched hearing loss is preventable just by wearing noise-deadening ear protection. For this reason, airport personnel exposed to high-pitched sounds of aircraft engines or municipal workers using a myriad of machinery should have ear protection in place.

Reaction Time: Or, If You Can't Be Quicker, Be Smarter

Your reflexes get slower as you age. But you knew that.

Studies among older people show that reaction latencies, or how fast we react, are slower than those for younger people. Also, the more complex the movements that are made, the greater the disparity in response latency with age.

Aging in general affects a wide variety of nonverbal information processing. A good example is trying to focus eyesight at distances after looking for a long time close-up. Fortunately, in older individuals, practice time still manages to shorten reaction time. Some geriatric facilities have even had success using Nintendo to sharpen mental acuity and hand-eye coordination of seniors.

A variable to consider when comparing the psychomotor performance of the young with the elderly—a 20 year old with a 70 year old, for example—is not just age. You also have to consider the dramatically different levels of health, physical fitness, and nutrition that individuals may have experienced during their lives. One study has shown how a four-month exercise program improved aerobic endurance and psychomotor performance in older athletes. The psychomotor latencies of older, physically fit men or women are shorter than those of sedentary individuals.

If you stay fit, you'll still inevitably end up losing quickness and reaction time, but you'll lose less of it.

That Mental Edge

In spite of the best efforts of your associates and family, you probably aren't losing your mind. Then why does it seem that as you get further into midlife, there are times when you're sure you are? In most instances, except in regard to the unfortunate progression of Alzheimer's disease, which knows no intellectual or personal fitness boundaries (but fortunately also afflicts fewer than one in five older adults), using the brain—like physical exercise—protects your memory and mental acuity. Studies also ascribe mental benefits for the elderly from three-times-a-week strength training. If this sounds very much like that Hellenic ideal of a sound mind and sound body, you're getting my drift.

The fact is that at any stage in life—but especially at midlife—cognitive problems are seldom caused by actual neural degeneration or change. They are most often due to other factors. There continues to be a considerable underappreciation of how depression and anxiety can interfere with cognition. Being depressed, stressed, anxious, or under some other mental pressure can masquerade as a loss of mental capacity. Commonly, such conditions might make you forgetful or distracted or interfere with your attention span.

Stress and confusion can turn into Edgar Allan Poe's "Descent into a Maelstrom." Depression and distraction can affect your performance on the job. Your wife and family can become upset with you. Your friends may try to avoid you. The whole process becomes a vicious cycle, with the effects exacerbating the condition, the condition creating still more deleterious effects, and so on. This, coupled with the other pressures associated with hitting midlife, can bring the enjoyment of life to a wicked halt. The worse it gets, the less able you're going to be to break the cycle.

Many men deal with this through self-medication—drugs or alcohol, to be specific. This creates still another complication, one from which society suffers greatly. Where does it all end?

Men, unlike women, don't go to the doctor or hospital unless they think they're dying. Women go for birth control pills, pap smears, babies, premarin (a hormone treatment for menopause), and so on. Their mothers have done this before them. But men have historically sought medical help only in acute situations, and sometimes not even then. If men don't seek medical help for an aching joint or even to get new glasses, how would they be expected to ask for assistance for something as nebulous as "mental illness"?

Fortunately, mental illness—or even just feeling blue, a bit out of sorts, less than top-notch—is increasingly being regarded more as a physical disease and less as something one can control through willpower: It's chemical, it's biological. There is a curious intermix among the workings of the brain, the body, and the spirit—one that we will probably never define—but just because you believe in the strength of one over the other doesn't mean you can't ask for help in areas where you are weak. That's what being a member of society is all about.

Thus, if you feel you may be losing your mind, a trip to the doc's could more easily solve a problem that could only get worse. An antidepressant drug or mood stabilizer, or simply just a few good conversations about what's on your mind, could break the stress cycle just enough to let you get back on task.

Don't let feeling down go too long. A good rule of thumb is: If someone tells you to seek help, they're probably right.

SUGGESTED READING

The PDR Family Guide to Prescription Drugs. Random House, 1996. 752 pp.

/ profile \

Dave Paulson

A Sport for All Seasons

Like a lot of men who decided right around the time they were fighting off pimples that they would lead an active life, Dave Paulson began his lifelong exercise program at age 13. That was when he was growing up in a small Minnesota town, easily missed if you blinked an eye going through it. However, there was an ample amount of Minnesota prairie for a boy to explore, hundreds of miles of the Minnesota River in which to drop a fish line, and an endless ribbon of country roads for great biking on any hot summer afternoon.

For Dave, traditional sports did not offer immediate success. "I spent five years at football practice and five years sitting on the bench," he says. "But at least I made it through all those years without an injury." Where Paulson did excel was cross-country. In college, he ran track and played tennis and soccer. At age 50-something, Dave's present regimen is laid-back in comparison with his earlier years. One summer when he was a high school teacher, he left for a two-and-a-half month canoe trip across Canada covering nine different river systems.

Dave currently plays tennis five days a week, works out on Nautilus three days, and either bikes, runs, or in-line skates another three days a week. "I'm on too many tennis leagues and teams. That's how I spend most of my money," he says. When winter arrives, he hits the cross-country ski trails at least every other day.

A picture hangs in Dave's wood frame Lake Minnetonka cottage of him hurling forward in classic cross-country style on the poster advertising the first Twin Cities Loppet ski race. Unfortunately, the race was canceled because of lack of snow. His first wife, behind him in the original poster, was airbrushed out by his sister.

At 6'1", Dave now weighs in the mid-180s, only 25 pounds more than he weighed at the end of high school, when he was also three inches shorter. Married and divorced twice—his first wife greeted him with divorce papers on his return from his Canadian canoe trip—Dave now with a soul mate, Meg, is the father of two grown boys. Dave and Meg relish traveling north to his splendid cabin in the tiny town of Cornucopia on the south shore of Lake Superior—an area unequaled for mountain biking, sailing, and cross-country skiing.

Dave's philosophy for healthy living is as unfancy as his Midwestern, down-to-earth lifestyle.

On food: "If teeth can bite it, I'll eat it," Dave says. About the only foods he avoids are processed items such as margarine, artificial sweetener, and artificial colors. "But if it's a fat, a vegetable, milk, potato, or bread, I'll eat it." Overall, Dave consumes about 5,500 to 6,000 calories a day. Snacking is okay, including a candy bar from time to time. "For me, I know when I'm out of shape and when I need to shape up," like when he was in divinity school and was pushing 194. But, he says, "Handball took the weight off real fast, about 20 pounds in eight months."

On staying in shape: "It's always easier to stay in shape than to have to try getting back into shape. The only real way to make it work," he says, "is to make it part of your lifestyle."

On growing old: "The folks who are waking up in the morning aching all over or are 25 pounds overweight find they can't do what they used to. Fortunately, I'm not experiencing these kinds of problems. My elbow or shoulder may hurt a little, but all I do is take a couple aspirins before I go out and play tennis." Aging, he says, "is mostly in the mind."

All this comes from a guy who never admits to all the tennis tournaments he has taken. But he will coyly admit that his biggest victory as an athlete came in two consecutive weekends in the early 1970s. In the first, he captured 10th place in the Mora Minnesota 58K Vasaloppet. In the second, he earned 50th out of 1,000 in the World Series of cross-country ski races, the North American Birkebeiner.

So while Dave's career has moved from teaching to educational computer sales, he's always found time for fitness. Whether it's tennis, running, bicycling, in-line skating, or skiing, he knows exactly what he'll be doing for the remaining decades of his life.

Chapter 4

On Slowing Down
■ It's the Masters, Not the Olympics

> Growing old is no more than a bad habit which a busy man has no time to form.
>
> André Maurois, *The Aging American*

Okay, this is the truth: Sorry to tell you, guys, but... Aging is a heterogeneous, genetically determined set of processes.

There simply aren't a whole lot of things we can do about it. That's the bad news. The good news is that despite all the signs our bodies show and the messages we get that we are aging, the slowing process does not have to be as dire as many of us fear. Some of the world's best over-40 master athletes prove that the older athlete may be able to keep up with his younger competitors—or at least keep them in sight—especially in the endurance sports.

Examples abound: The marathon in the 1984 Olympics was won by 37-year-old Carlos Lopes. In cross-country skiing—arguably the most aerobically demanding sport of all—the Olympic 1988 silver medal in the men's 50-kilometer race was taken by 39-year-old Maurilio DeZolt of Italy, who repeated the feat in 1992 at age 43! He then finished in the top 10 in that event in Lillehammer in 1994.

So biological aging alone may not be the limiting factor in how well one man runs the marathon. Besides the obvious factor—dedicated conditioning—such intangibles as job stress, inevitable hassles with children, or an aging parent suddenly diagnosed with lung cancer can have a significant impact.

Still, there are enough changes in our lives and especially in our physical capacity to make us question whether we can still leap over the fence in pursuit of an errant four year old. Is this an indication of some irreversible, age-induced disability? Maybe. Maybe not.

Here, to the best of my ability, is the latest rundown on what your aging body can or cannot do, assuming that you maintain a modicum of fitness and health.

Is It Age, or Have I Always Been This Way?

Age does provoke a wide array of functions (and dysfunctions). We aren't as quick. We aren't as strong. Our joints may not move as easily or as far. Some other body parts (many of which we've already discussed in previous chapters) degenerate, stiffen up, or generally don't work as well. The late S. J. Perelman described the condition with humor and insight in his book *Under the Spreading Atrophy.* We wish it were, but aging is not always a humorous or simple matter. Physical function can still be preserved to a great extent by careful attention to your body. Physical conditioning, reduction of stress, a good diet, and a host of other intercessions can hold off the decline and in some cases even reverse it. In plain English, If you don't use it, you lose it. Following a plan of regularly scheduled maintenance should keep you running right.

We've been conditioned to accept a certain amount of dysfunction as we age. Yet it doesn't have to be that way. We love the story, for example, of the elderly patient who goes to see his doctor. Doctor Cohen examines his sore right leg and says, "I'm not surprised that you have some problems with your leg. You're not a youngster any more. You're almost 80." The annoyed patient retorts, "But Doc, my left leg's 80 too, and it doesn't hurt."

The point is that there definitely are preconceptions and misconceptions about growing older. For instance, some would have us believe that we aren't supposed to do certain things any longer because we are aging, or that our bodies have inexorably deteriorated and there's nothing we can do about it. These, it appears, are myths. Thank the gods. Just think of Roy Carlsted, an internationally ranked ski racer who at 70 keeps up joyfully with racers 30 years his junior (laughing at them, to boot, as he speeds by).

Muscle Strength, or Can I Still Impress Girls at the Beach?

As you age, your muscles lose strength. If you are active, if you exercise and participate in sports, that loss will be minimized. But if you insist on being a couch potato, watch out! Those precious muscles will get noticeably flabbier and weaker. And you're going to have a tough time getting to the refrigerator. But you probably figured this slice of reality out already.

Muscle strength is defined as the maximum force (tension) generated by a muscle in a single maximal (read "all-out") contraction. Just as there is a loss of muscle strength, there is also a decrease in muscle mass with aging, commensurate with a decline in the size and number of your muscle fibers. Such an inevitable decline, however, is smaller among active older adults (like my friend Roy). Naturally, this decline is a function of the type of activity you choose and how the muscles are used. Evidence suggests that vigorous activity, such as weight lifting, running or swimming intervals, pace workouts, and racing, can actually reverse this muscle loss (maybe, so much for a very mellow jog three times a week). In fact, older men (and women too) can actually increase their maximum strength by exactly the same percentage as younger subjects, but only after just eight weeks of progressive strength training. In short, exercise can have as beneficial—and as immediate—an effect on an older body as on a younger one. Hey, guys, that means you.

Endurance: If You Can't Do It As Well, at Least You Can Do It Longer

For those who participate in endurance sports, there is even more to be cheerful about. There is less loss of the endurance capacity that sustains us in a marathon than there is of the muscle strength that counts so heavily in an anaerobic event such as a sprint. Read on.

Endurance is defined as the capacity of the body to sustain while performing continuous submaximal contractions—that is, maintaining a less than all-out pace for an extended period of time. This is why many runners, swimmers, cyclists, or cross-country skiers gravitate toward longer races as they age. Such a progression is testimony to how endurance predominates over strength as we age. We may not be faster, but at least we can go longer.

When age-related changes in athletes over 30 are reviewed, running speed of men over 40 declines less with longer races than with shorter races as compared with similar times for younger athletes. This difference is substantiated by microscopic changes found in our neurons as well as at the muscle, tendon, and cartilage level. Strength (speed) losses are greater than endurance losses, and results in the sprint are more likely to decline with age than in the marathon. Losses are also greater in events such as high, long, and triple jumps, where explosive strength becomes a more significant factor.

One theory, by the way, on why older men perform better at longer races is that many opt to avoid rigorous, intense, and often painful interval training required for the shorter length races (I know that as I entered my late forties, I certainly did). In other words, although they are able to compete in shorter events, they often choose not to. As the body changes, so does the mind, or maybe vice versa.

With years (should) come(s) wisdom.

VO$_{max}$

One convenient measure of aerobic fitness is called the VO$_{max}$. It is essentially a measurement of the maximum amount of oxygen a person can use per minute per kilogram of body weight. It typically declines 1 percent each year past age 25.

However, if the amount of physical activity and body composition is kept constant, the decline can be minimized to less than 0.05 percent a year. Keeping in mind that mind and body are interrelated, a decline in VO_{max} is not just age related, but influenced by other factors, such as age at onset of training, how much you train, any history of illness, or your genetic profile—the parents you didn't choose.

Effective training can prove effective time and again in maintaining and improving physical fitness. A 1987 evaluation of 24 male track athletes ages 50 to 82 reported the effect of age in training on VO_{max} over 10 years. Those who remained active maintained a 10 percent higher VO_{max} than their noncompetitive cohorts even though each group showed the same decline in maximum heart rate (there are certain things over which we have no control).

Keep in mind that the majority of the general population wouldn't run for a bus. Most aging men must accept that they are, unfortunately, slowing down in a few more ways than one. But you don't have to let the reality of your aging affect you all that drastically. Sure, you may lose speed, but you don't have to lose endurance. So, all in all, as we cruise through our forties and into our fifties, we have to expect some decline in strength, and an expected decline in the speed we are capable of achieving. Adaptation is the message here. That there seems to be less decline in endurance activities explains why older athletes can achieve some impressive results in endurance events.

Most loss in aerobic capacity fortunately is something that can be controlled by an act of will (mind and body again). You can *will* yourself to stay physically fit and make that conscious decision part of your daily regimen. But although the Olympics may be out of the question, statistics confirm you can maintain body (and mind?) if you exercise reasonably and remain fit. Rather than sprinting into your forties only to fizzle out at this critical turning point, the idea, I believe, is to keep at it for the rest of your life. Albeit, as you motor along, you're ultimately gonna be shuffling along. But that's really OK.

SUGGESTED READINGS

Caine, K. Winston. *The Male Body: An Owner's Manual.* St. Martin's Press, 1996. 405 pp.

Reichel, William. *Clinical Aspects of Aging.* Williams and Wilkins, 1983. 642 pp.

Rybeck, David, MD. *Look Ten Years Younger. Live Ten Years Longer: A Man's Guide.* Rodale Press, 1995. 318 pp.

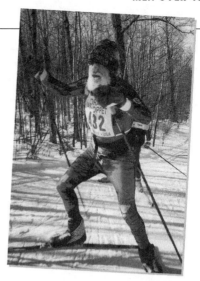

Roy Carlsted

Aging Actively

It had been a fine Minnesota cross-country ski day—20 degrees Fahrenheit, winter sun dogs in the sky, crisp powder on a hard track—when Roy, my ski buddy, and I realized we were lost. We had driven two hours north from Minneapolis to Kathio State Park near Lake Milaca, and there was no one out in the woods except plenty of nervous deer and us. The sky showed that dusk was setting in; we had three hours of hard skiing behind us and were running pretty much on empty.

I knew I had a half an hour and maybe a little to spare before hypothermia might set in. That's when you don't make sense anymore—a body temperature of 90°F (32°C) can be an ominous sign.

This was a few years ago, when Roy Carlsted was a mere youngster at age 68. Fitness-minded year-round, he took in three 40-minute workouts a week. Even with this modest amount of exercise, he sported the oxygen consumption of a sedentary man 40 years his junior. He was the classic demonstration that the quality of our years can be enhanced by following a prescription of moderate lifelong activity for the high-risk and healthy alike.

Back in the woods, we both stopped to collect ourselves. The worst thing you can do in a situation like ours is to panic. We'd been trading leads for most of the afternoon, critiquing each other's style in the classic cross-country, or diagonal, technique. This means we push off one arm and thrust the opposite ski forward with a tempo that makes our bodies glide smoothly along the trail—a delightful marriage of style, equipment, and training.

The sky wasn't any help, a typical overcast midwinter Minnesota late afternoon. There was no setting sun to use for direction. Working now as a survival team, we decided to try to pick up speed and make a sincere effort to find our way on the snow-covered park road. We knew it had to go to ,or come from, someplace. I began to feel my panic lift as I watched my companion, some 20 years older than I, skate to and fro on our route to freedom. At last we began to recognize the trail back to the warming house.

"Ten minutes of body heat left," I thought, knowing I was dehydrated and, without a shell over my lycra ski suit, in danger of losing too much body heat to the ominously cooling day.

Roy, a farm boy by birth, turned to this urban doctor, smiled, and said reassuringly, "We'll be back in five minutes. Try to sink your pole a little further forward. The secret is hanging out as far as you can on the gliding ski."

Simple, I thought. Here I had been thinking about survival. Roy reminded me that it was just one step—one glide—at a time.

Chapter 5

The Psychology of Aging

■ Midlife Opportunity

Old age isn't so bad when you consider the alternative.

Maurice Chevalier, *New York Times,* Oct. 9, 1960

Here's looking at you. Have you ever noticed that actually, the person you see when you peer into the bathroom mirror with partially closed eyes seems very little different from that guy you remember in college? Maybe this is some inner method of decreasing the pain of the reality of getting older staring back at you. While driving, you glance up at your rearview mirror and discover more white hairs growing from your temples. "Oh heck," you rationalize, "I look so distinguished with gray hair around my temples. So my hairline is receding. Who's perfect?"

The psychology of aging has been well documented by James Birren and Warner Schaie in the *Handbook of the Psychology of Aging* (4th ed., Academic Press, 1996). That the first *Handbook of the Psychology of Aging* was published 28 years after the first *Handbook of Child Psychology* tells you a lot about our societal priorities. Or is it the fact that the largest segment of our population is now 85? After all, at the time *Child Psychology* was printed, the fastest growing segment of the population was the baby boom generation. Now, it's over 85! In turn, societal priorities may evolve accordingly.

But societal respect does not necessarily lead to statistical prominence. Even today, in spite of all the stories in the news about the significance of older adults, studies show that physicians actually spend significantly less time with nursing-home patients (often, mere seconds) than with middle-aged, office-based patients. In the ongoing debate on health care, any proposed "rationing" of medical procedures seems to favor younger people because they rank higher on the priority list than older people. The very elderly, and especially the institutionalized aged, frequently become not only everyone's burden but superfluous. I am, however, more than a little surprised by the age of one or another older patient who gets a coronary bypass or carotid angioplasty in his or her late seventies or eighties.

My own mother underwent quadruple bypass two or three years before her death at 71 although she was on dialysis. Yet her operation gave her time and the strength to cope with the end.

Such aspects of aging could certainly lead to a certain amount of understandable stress and anxiety…if we let them. At 40, potentially with more years behind us than ahead of us, reality can start to sink in…if we let it. Our forties and beyond can be considerably worrisome as we face our own mortality. We can also find ourselves caught between the Scylla of aging parents and the Charybdis of rambunctious, acting-out adolescents, with the siren song of a midlife crisis on the horizon.

If this isn't scary, then you just aren't alive, man.

Stress Is Bad for You

Stress is a classic example of the interaction between body and mind, the physical and the mental. Your mind may perceive a threat of some kind, and your body reacts by secreting hormones to help you deal with the threat. Some have called this process the "fight or flight" response because ages ago, when our bodies first evolved, the process of stress was normally a response to a life-or-death situation. Making the right choice between fight or flight could literally be a matter of your survival.

The hormones in question are substances such as adrenaline. They tend to hop you up and increase your physical capacity. If you respond physically, the hormones are used up. If you vegetate, as is unfortunately often the lot of modern desk jockeys, the hormones can just build up, possibly consuming you from the inside.

Amid the happy talk about the wonderful things you can do to improve your life in your forties and beyond, there is no denying that you are getting older, not younger. Though I'm not suggesting your lives won't change with age, I suggest that there are ways to cope with anxiety to really make those years challenging and fun.

Recent research done on stress suggests that the threat from too much unresolved mental turmoil may be even greater than we realized. Although most people realize that ulcers could be one result of too much stress, few are truly aware of the effects of stress on "killer cells"—vital components in the blood that float around like free-lance bodyguards. If they see something they don't like—something they perceive as foreign to the body—they "kill" it. This includes cancer cells. Cancer can begin as a single aberrant cell or as a few abnormal cells that start to grow in an out-of-control manner. Killer cells discover these cells and try to off them. Some experts theorize that this happens in the human body all the time, and that only on rare occasions do cancer cells grow enough to cause trouble.

The problem is that stress, according to these theories, depresses killer cell activity, thus reducing your ability to fend off disease and, potentially, one big meltdown.

Family Pressure

Usually, you get home late and are totally whipped. More often than not, you are a two-income family and need every penny of it. Your wife arrives at about the same time you do, probably having beaten the closing of day care by only minutes (though that's just as likely the dad's job these days), and she's as toasted as you are. It quickly becomes evident that you can't expect her to perform the support services for the family that your mother supplied for your father.

With or without kids, you have to put food on the table. So you slap down the easiest, fastest thing you can find. It is not coincidental that there has been a proliferation of fast-food restaurants everywhere. (There are at least 60 McDonald's restaurants each in New York City and Istanbul.) Only on rare occasions can junk food be considered healthy. In addition to everything else is the realization that you're getting older and feeling bad about that, too.

CAVEAT

We baby boomers can be forgiven for believing that some evil deity has deliberately chosen our lifetimes in which to throw our world into chaos. Any innocent preconceptions we may have had about how our lives would unfold have been turned upside down, leaving us challenged to make the new rules work.

And it feels as if the screenplay has sometimes been written cruelly and deceptively. Think about it.

We were the ones who grew up in the fifties, immersed in the four-square Republican ideal of How Life Should Be. Dad had a job, we owned a house, and Mom provided support while remaining eternally cheerful (do I hear shades of June Cleaver here?). Well, it turned out not like that for us kids. So what happened?

There has been a significant decline in our earning power. Not only must we have two incomes per household just to break even, but our employers are often able to demand that we work longer hours for less pay (adjusted for inflation). Meanwhile, as costs go up for health care and retirement planning, benefits mysteriously go down. Haven't you wondered at the number of independent contractors and temps holding down many of the jobs at one big bank or another (they do not qualify for benefits).

To try to make more money, many boomers change jobs every several years or so. I've joked with friends that I change jobs more than most people change underwear. We've often been told by the self-help gurus, "Your best raise is your starting salary." But does this ploy actually work? Your guess is as good as mine. Whereas our parents and grandparents worked for years for the same company, our boss thinks nothing of tossing us into the street to extend the almighty profit margin, not to mention his annual bonus. I have found that my well-being as an employee was of little significance compared to that of the corporation.

Guess who gets the ax first? (1) The guy with the least tenure, or (2) the older guy who earns too much money. In either case, *we do.* Generation X is just a few steps behind and waiting in the wings to do the same job for less. (A note on their behalf: Economically, it hasn't been fun and games for them, either. Nor will it change in the foreseeable future.) The long-range effect is that we never seem to stay in place long enough to vest a pension. That, too, may be part of the company plan. I just learned that a friend who was the upper-school headmaster of a prominent local prep school for a decade of his 30-year teaching tenure left for first one then a second exciting temporary job. At the time of his mysterious suicide in Cairo, he had no life insurance to maintain his widow.

Why?

Midlife Crisis and You

While we're on the subject of suicide, it does seem that almost daily a name leaps out at you from the obituary page: acquaintances, friends, classmates, heroes, enemies. This is just one of the many ways that you can be reminded of your own mortality—a conclusion to life you never bothered to consider in your immortal youth. Living in a culture that worships youth at the expense of the "golden agers" doesn't help. Early-twentieth-century philosopher and educator John Dewey once said that "we are at present more or less in the unpleasant and illogical condition of extolling maturity and deprecating age." Such an ethos seems to be more and more true when we consider the current image of aging.

Just watch television. Situation comedy, which has often parodied stupid ethnics, subservient women, and comic homosexuals, also portrays older people as out-of-touch, doddering fools fond of retelling the same boring stories and barely able to keep from wetting their pants. Whatever happened to the time when older people were valued for their experience and wisdom?

Fortunately, this perception has been improving. Despite our once famous cry, "Never trust anyone over 30," we suddenly realize that, "Oh my God, this is us now!" Yes, the sheer weight of numbers of the maturing baby boomers has forced society to make that accommodation to age. It shows up in the form of fashion models with lines on their faces, replacing prepubescent types of 20 years ago. I found it interesting to see the lone older male model in a local clothing company's catalogue, dressed for his 30th reunion but unquestionably with a 20-year younger trophy significant other in tow. Rock 'n roll tours are populated now by graying heroes we'd have sworn would have overdosed long ago. They're too smart for that. They'd rather make millions and invest in mutual funds. Even Ozzie Osbourne, whom I saw not long ago, has come a long way, baby, from biting chickens' heads off.

Is anybody out there truly happy about getting old? Of course not. But things do go better if we deal with the reality of aging openly and knowledgeably.

What Are Your Concerns?

There are endless permutations of things to be concerned about as you age—that is, if you decide to spend your time perseverating about them. If you do so, you can create your own particular and personalized blend of angst.

In general, the problem could seem to revolve around loss. You can let yourself be concerned that you're becoming less than what you once were—less capable, less attractive, less able to compete. You may face what you perceive as a diminution in your capacity—you worry you may be slower, weaker, or (heaven forbid!) duller. You may even fear you're not worth talking to. Like invisible. On the other hand, of course, there's that mythology: rich is sexy, and there's a pretty good chance that you're financially comfortable as you pass through your forties.

Once, being older meant being possessed of the accumulated wisdom of society. Elders were sought out in times of trouble and were not regarded as people to be avoided. Paleolithic clans relied on the older men to provide the locations of safe trails, good shelter, hunting secrets, and spiritual incantations. Just think back to democratic Athens, where elders dominated the vote. Coups to unseat them from power or financial reward were nonexistent.

Let's get back to the loss issue: The concerns of someone at midlife predominantly seem to revolve around mental deterioration. You know you're losing hair and muscle mass and that young women aren't noticing you any more—other than to be very polite and open the door for you. You feel you're losing your capacity, your attractiveness, even your mind. You've been bombarded by information telling you that somehow you'll become mentally less sharp as you get older. I know, at 53, I am more than a little paranoid when I can't remember a name. Am I losing my marbles?

The good news, at least where your mind is concerned, is that it doesn't have to be that way. Despite the pressures of life, your mind will remain as alert as it was 10 to 20 years earlier. Some temporary diminishment can be expected but doesn't have to be prolonged. A bout of anxiety about taxes, the loss of a relative, money woes, a lover, a job, or a child can sometimes produce confusion, incoherence, or despondency. It's no secret that the worries and the stress of midlife can result in anxiety and depression.

We are, as John Dewey pronounced, "increasingly wise and mature while at the same time increasingly biologically vulnerable and likely to die." As Jim Morrison said, "No one gets out of here alive."

Eliminate the Physical

Chapter 3 covered neurological changes in midlife. Whether we like it or not, psychological and physiological aspects of behavior are inextricably interlinked. One does not exist without the other. Because the physiological is far easier to quantify than the psychological, it is always best to look to the body first for a cause of mental breakdown. The following paragraphs survey some physical conditions that can masquerade as psychological ones. If they prove treatable, your troubles may be ended.

Heredity

One area worth watching is an emerging discipline of developmental behavioral genetics (hereditary causes of behavior). Central to this field is the notion that one-third to one-half of most behavioral differences may be due to genetic causes. A gene on chromosome 21, for example, has been implicated in some cases of familially transmitted Alzheimer's disease. However, this still leaves most of the variance attributable to non-genetic causes. This further emphasizes the need to consider environmental reasons for individual differences as a function of aging.

Dementia

There are many illnesses—60, to be exact—that can cause dementia. Although medical reporters on the evening news like to give you the impression that Alzheimer's disease is virtually inevitable, the fact is that only 6 percent of all dementia in seniors can be attributed to Alzheimer's. Ten to 20 percent of people who have dementia may have an underlying (possibly reversible) systemic medical disorder, such as liver or kidney disease, which is treatable. Other etiologies, such as metabolic imbalances or drug interactions, are not only preventable but, fortunately, reversible.

IS IT REAL, OR IS IT MEMORY?

There are always the horror stories about seniors thought to be "out of it," only to make a miraculous recovery after someone discovered they were overmedicated or that their eyeglasses or hearing aids had been lost for two months. This is far more common than we'd like to believe, especially among the very elderly.

For example, a friend recently visited his 98-year-old, nursing-home-bound, nearly blind and deaf grandmother and was alarmed to find her staring blankly into space. After trying for a while to get some coherent response from her, his sister replaced grandma's hearing aid batteries. She looked up as if awakening and said very clearly, "That's better. Can we begin our conversation again, please?"

Though the body is weak, the mind is just fine, thank you.

Reversible causes of dementia include infectious diseases, metabolic problems, and even occult hydrocephalus—literally, "water on the brain" —a condition in which cerebrospinal fluid in one of the cerebral ventricles gets blocked, swelling the ventricle and compressing the brain.

Dementia can be hard to cope with once it arrives, but it often is detectable by a very thorough clinical evaluation, or by avoiding indiscriminate self-medication or oversedation in an older patient. Dementia is less a disease than it is a collection of symptoms. It has causes, and where there are causes, there is a chance of prevention. Much of that prevention can happen now, not at age 65.

Preventive measures should be considered even if you suspect that you or your loved one may have Alzheimer's disease (AD). AD is not all that common, and of those people who do have it, a sizable percentage suffer from complications such as stroke and heart disease, which make the dementia progress more quickly. Here's where prevention makes so much sense. Statistically, the best candidates for dementia, with or without Alzheimer's disease, are individuals between the ages of 50 and 65 with a history of high blood pressure or diabetes—both of which, if not preventable, are certainly controllable through diet, exercise, and proper health care.

You can do a great deal with your lifestyle to decrease morbidity and mortality from dementia. Age, sex, and family history remain independent variables—that is, there is very little any of you can do about the parents and grandparents you inherited. But you may be able to reduce certain biological risk factors through a simple act of will, by eliminating them from your lifestyle. These include smoking, excessive alcohol consumption, Type A behavior patterns, ambient hostility, job strain, psychosocial stress, or factors contributing to sexual malfunction. Some members of the health care community even consider strokes borderline self-inflicted illnesses. If you associate hypertension with strokes, then this assumption may not be far off the mark.

The point is that before you assume you've contracted some deep-seated mental disorder, you should first consider that you're suffering from a physical (and potentially curable) condition that only indirectly affects your mind.

Actual Psychological Problems at Midlife

Now for the other head problems. Physiological problems aside, simply being in midlife, with the attendant stressors and physical changes to deal with, could cause plenty of mental anguish. A percentage of your angst, however, may be plenty difficult, if not downright impossible, to do anything about. You could, of course, make it a practice to watch funny movies several times a week and get in your daily quota of belly laughs.

Take the rampant youth reversion that some midlifers tend to fall into, including chasing around after forbidden sexual adventures. This process can easily destroy a family—yours, to be specific, and perhaps hers too. Let's face it, if you're feeling old, fat, and unloved, and some attentive younger woman suddenly seems turned on by your presence, it's going to be hard to remember how much you love and respect your wife. Most of us can actually do it (don't believe everything you see on *Knott's Landing),* but you're only human when other less human thoughts cross your mind. Fortunately, most men can still prioritize their passions.

In addition to adultery, or whatever you decide to call your particular transgression, there are any number of other manifestations of midlife change. They range from fad diets to running off to Sturgis, South Dakota, on a motorcycle with your dental hygienist. And midlife changes can cause some pretty aberrant behavior, too—a sudden need for a divorce, quitting your job or changing your profession, beginning the cocktail hour at 10 o'clock in the morning, and purchasing outrageously expensive or possibly dangerous motorized toys (my single 50-year-old plastic surgeon friend arrived at my house the other day on his Valkyrie motorcycle—the longest motorcycle made—on his way to take his plane up for a flight). Talk about phallic extensions.

I'm not going to get into long, deep discussions about the wisdom of buying a sensible family car instead of the low-slung sports job that you think you need. It's your life, and more or less 50 percent of it is your money, depending on which state you live in. There are, however, pressing problems that afflict many of us that must be dealt with intelligently and, often, immediately.

Depression and Suicide

According to Albert Camus, there is only one truly philosophical question, and that is suicide. Hamlet would have agreed (and he wasn't even near 40, despite the maturity of all the actors who have played him in the twentieth century). Like dementia, the desire to terminate your life is a behavioral symptom that may be linked to more than one problem, frequently occurring as a part of major depression, alcoholism, or schizophrenia.

Statistics confirm that aging has at least a circumstantial relationship with suicide, with the rate highest in the 65 and over age group. Suicide is 25 percent more common among white males age 65 to 74 compared with those who are 18 to 24, and over 70 percent more common among white males age 75 to 84 compared to the 18- to 24-year-old group. It is often difficult to tell just how much "disguised" forms of suicide—those that are simply not reported—inflate these statistics. One person may leave a lengthy suicide note, and another may jump off a building (both fairly obvious). Another may simply get drunk and drive his car into a bridge abutment (hard to tell). In the latter instances, the causes we often accept are "icy road," "falling asleep while driving," or "DWI." The truth may be more like, "fed up with life, family, job, self." But the ultimate response is, "what a sorrowful thing to do for you and for us."

I realize this is to be a positive book to help you become or maintain vigorousness through your forties. The message: Don't kill yourself, because those you punish are your loved ones. Despite multiple causes, the common denominator of suicidal depression can be summarized in one phrase: Those who commit suicide share a belief that their lives are no longer worth living. Why, we ask, should people feel that way more strongly as they age?

Illness certainly can play a part. Very few people in old age are well one moment and dead the next. Death can be a long, drawn-out process, and a terminal or debilitating illness is more the norm than not. In these instances, depression may not always be a factor in suicide. Some people, most notably members of the Hemlock Society, matter-of-factly decide to exercise the one control over the universe that they believe they must always self-determine: whether they live or die. This is where Camus's observation applies. Yet because most very ill people generally prefer to hope for recovery and live, this belief is certainly not universal. I have personally struggled with why someone with the most bleak cancer would be willing to risk nausea, no white count, and infection on the slim chance he could live. Perhaps this is the human condition.

Depression is another matter, and largely a function of one's emotional profile. Depression clouds thinking and leads to indecision, low self-esteem, paranoia, feelings of worthlessness, and often thoughts of death. Depressed behavior varies widely, but it can often worsen with heavy drinking. (After all, alcohol is a depressant.) Maybe we need to take another look at the motivation behind driving while intoxicated, irrational risk taking, or destructive and even senseless marital infidelity. What these behaviors have in common is an uncontrollable urge for self-destruction either directed at oneself or at one's relationships. It's almost a perverse willingness to tear apart your life.

How serious is the prospect of depression as you get older? Studies show that nearly 25 percent of elderly men seen by doctors for physical health problems also have symptoms of depression. Another study has suggested that five out of nine older men with gastrointestinal problems may have underlying psychological problems. Out of 300 persons with gastrointestinal difficulties, 56 percent (compared with 44 percent from physical factors) had GI pain from psychological causes. These included irritable colon, spastic colitis, gastritis, heartburn, nausea, diarrhea, and constipation. This leaves us to reconsider the old chicken-and-the-egg routine: To what extent is depression causing physical ailments, and to what extent could it be the other way around?

How prone are men to dysphoria, that emotion between "the blues" and abject depression? It's often hard to say. On the one hand, a macho nature frequently forbids men from talking about their despondency, let alone beginning to deal with it. It is commonly held, because they are more vocal about their emotions, that women suffer more from depression than men. But do we believe that just because women are more prone to express their difficulties? Keep in mind the old saw that when it comes to attempting suicide, "Women try, men do." Too many men never communicate their pain until it is too late—after they have pulled the trigger, jumped from the window, or driven the car into a tree. A man's last exit unfortunately too often lacks any forewarning. Regardless, it is so terribly final.

Are women simply depressive "chickens?" Not really. The point could be argued either way. Obviously, the ability to cope and persevere should easily be seen as a stronger rational course. It is one thing to swallow a dozen sleepers as an attention-getting cry for help, but another to swallow the business end of a revolver under the influence of just enough of a depressant and disinhibitor such as alcohol.

Why, then, we wonder, do men seem to be more prone to such high-visibility difficulties during midlife? Men have certainly gotten quite a bit of press for their legendary midlife crises. One difference between the sexes may offer a clue. Men, as we've discussed, really struggle with a decrease in their perception of their physical powers, which they have been taught from birth (if not encoded in their genetic makeup) are vital for a meaningful life. Women, on the other hand, by midlife are just beginning to leave their childbearing years—an obvious time of weighty responsibility, if not actual physical danger. To many (though not all) women, leaving the procreative period may come not as a shock and cause for depression but rather as a huge relief. I've seen plenty of 40-year-old women setting out on their own personal journeys, often not in sync with the mate of the last 20 years.

Overall, women appear to register higher rates of psychiatric treatment for such narrowly defined mental illnesses as neurosis or functional psychoses, but not for the brain syndromes or personality disorders. When we find a woman sitting in a psychiatrist's waiting room, she is frequently there to deal with depression or unhappiness that she, at least, is willing to admit as her own. "Guy things" include aggression, physical abuse, or violent behavior, antisocial personality disorders, or alcohol and drug abuse. If a man is at the shrink's for treatment for any of these, it is often at the urging of his wife, a social worker, or a family counselor, or mandated by some local court. Are we bad boys again?

As we age, one reality we have to anticipate is that a depressed friend, loved one, business associate, or patient may come out of the haze of a deep depression just long enough to pull the trigger. What should have we done?

My friend Dan, an educator, moved to Cairo to start a new American-style secondary school after two less-than-successful jobs in the United States. For a while, I was hearing from him on a regular basis. Then the letters became less frequent. Several months later, we heard he was dead. He apparently hung himself in his apartment at the new school. No warning. No letter. No nothing.

Sensitivity, an open ear for warning signs in ourselves or our friends, and perhaps even a more pragmatic denial of the necessity for self-destruction are all options we need to keep in mind. We have to listen, react sensitively, and be aware enough to disarm our best friend's Smith and Wesson if he's in the vegetative blues. There may not be many hints to make our caring timely.

Economic Status and Stress

People at higher socioeconomic levels are generally in better health and have lower rates of disability and premature death. In comparison to the general population, African-Americans have a shortened life expectancy at birth and at all times in their life have more disability. They have a higher incidence of hypertension, cancer, coronary artery disease, cerebrovascular disease, diabetes, obesity, and higher crude mortality rates. They also face a far greater chance of dying by violent means than their Caucasian counterparts.

These disturbing realities show the effect of race and ethnicity as well as cross-cultural issues in any research on aging. Primarily, they emphasize the relationship between such physical stressors as a poverty lifestyle and later physical and mental health problems. African-Americans and other people of color may represent a disproportionately high percentage among those below the poverty line. They are also more likely to suffer such problems related to the stress of a poor lifestyle.

Sleep Disorders

As you age, it's not unusual to encounter more trouble sleeping. The problem can be with falling asleep, staying asleep, or simply the quality of your sleep. Lack of sleep can disrupt work and family life, bring about demotion or firing, create tension with your children, and even lead to divorce. Far more often than people realize, lack of sleep can cause accidents, particularly while you are driving, leading to disability or death. Unfortunately, a certain amount of sleep impairment may be inevitable with age. The quality of your sleep may deteriorate. Often you may experience increased nighttime wakefulness, and sleep becomes more fragmented. The older we are, the more easily we can be disturbed during sleep. We do not sleep as deeply and have a harder time staying asleep.

Yet sleep disorders do not necessarily have to be a normal part of aging. It is important to differentiate between psychological and physiological reasons for sleep problems. Early-morning wakening, so-called terminal insomnia, for example, can be one symptom of depression. Difficulty falling asleep, on the other hand, can be more a symptom of anxiety.

It really is too simplistic a solution to ask your physician to prescribe a drug such as Valium or Xanax (two popular benzodiazepams) or a hypnotic such as Restoril (excellent for insomnia and anxiety). Finding and dealing with the problem may make more sense over the long haul than blasting off the tip of an emotional iceberg with drugs, hoping it will melt away. Xanax can be an effective temporary bandage for people suffering from sleep deprivation and anxiety. Plenty of 40 year olds would probably be willing to delve into the painful reasons why their lives aren't working provided they can get just one good night's sleep. Your physician can prescribe a "sleeper" for you, hoping your depression and anxiety are self-limited—for example, from the death of a parent, an unexpected rejection in a relationship, or a professional setback. Fortunately, depression often is seasonal or limited to a month or so at a time. Nonetheless, should depression strike and hang on for more than a few weeks' time or should it constantly recur, you should see a health care professional experienced in dealing with such a condition. The good side of the story is that many dysphoric problems are biochemical and can be corrected with the right medication.

Again, the first step in dealing with sleep disorders is to eliminate any physical causes. There are some very logical medical reasons for certain sleep problems. Prostate enlargement with symptoms of urinary obstruction and subsequent overflow incontinence could be waking you up. It's not that you can't sleep, you just find you're getting up every hour to urinate. Or having rheumatoid arthritis can make any sleeping position you try painful. Also, if you have swollen, painful fingers or wrists or angry knee joints, it comes as no surprise that you may find sleep difficult.

Heart problems can be another reason for irregular sleep. For instance, a man with congestive heart failure could literally be drowning in his own body fluids, especially after lying down to go to sleep. He may describe the need to throw open the window for air. He could be suffering from swollen, even painful legs, also due to heart failure.

In any event, if you are having trouble sleeping, don't hesitate to seek medical help. With the calcium channel blockers, "-ase" inhibitors, and inotropic meds such as digitalis, there can be pharmaceutical solutions to your problems.

Anxiety and the Workplace

Another psychological affliction frequently seen among aging men is that grab bag of neuroses known as anxiety. Surprisingly, there are negligible differences in the amount of anxiety you experience with age, even though the causes may change.

Anxiety is characterized by feelings of tension, apprehension, with heightened autonomic nervous system activity. Translation: You get twitchy, sweaty, and fidgety, and you want to get away from whatever is making you frightened.

There are many obvious sources for anxiety as you pass 40. Work, family, and money are three major causes, but there are also fears about aging, impending retirement, and even death. Sadly, much of the anxiety of aging is founded in reality. Ours is very much a youth-oriented society, and men are not being overly paranoid when they fear that they can easily be replaced at work by someone younger. This is not altogether different from the societal behavior in much of the animal world, which constantly pits the up-and-coming young males against the aging group leaders.

Women of late have been telling us that we have only ourselves to blame, that much of what is the "corporate style" is typically male. They mean that in the male-dominated workplace, most relationships and managerial styles are still founded on male competitiveness. Women, they tell us, might give the older worker another role more suited to his or her condition and talent. Young women are known to change the rules in an effort to maintain friendships. Theirs is a philosophy of compromise and accommodation to preserve relationships, sometimes at all costs.

There is no easy answer here. As individuals, we may be unable to overcome such epidemic age discrimination, especially one with so compelling an economic reinforcement. The short-term individual solution is for each of us to be constantly vigilant to the worst-case scenario that could befall our career. In other words, planning is important, yet anticipation is all.

Anxiety frequently has its basis in feelings of powerlessness. You could discover that you are not in the best position at your job. As you get older, you may discover that wrinkles, arthritic knees, hypertension, and cancer can work as a disadvantage for you in the workplace. Denying it can only cause you more anxiety.

For that reason alone, your forties are a logical time to decide what you intend to do when you "grow up." You are still young enough to have considerable room to maneuver in the workplace. You also have a fair share of knowledge about what's likely to happen in that arena—you've been bloodied a bit in combat, and you know the ropes. Start by considering what effects age might eventually have on your career. This one is up for grabs. A lot has to do with a patient's personal preference: Marcus Welby or George Clooney. All factors being equal, both cognitive and procedural skills should stay constant. There's much to be said for increasing experience with years of practice. If you're a professional football player, you'd better have a lifeboat available (orange parachute acceptable), usually by your late twenties. Then again, making more than $1 million a year makes early retirement sound better all the time.

If you do hard physical labor, now might be the time to take that course necessary to become a project supervisor. If you're a logger who makes his living cutting trees where environmentalists have discovered endangered species, you might consider night school in an entirely different field. This may seem like pretty basic stuff. But failure to plan ahead can further contribute to feelings of helplessness and impotence, literally and figuratively.

Anxiety and the Bedroom

Then there's the other anxiety—women. Turning 40 may mean you could become invisible to women under 25. But maybe that's for the better; it keeps you from getting in trouble. And even if this doesn't bother you, there is still that current relationship to maintain.

Diminishing physical abilities often create anxiety related to sex. Sadly, there are plenty of us who fail to recognize what's going on in our marriages or relationships until they get stressed to the breaking point. The central dilemma is usually not about sex at all. This is perhaps why so many men who seek to recapture lost youth in various sexual adventures may still love and feel attracted to their wives, current or estranged. They're stepping out for other reasons.

Perhaps this behavior is akin to "bathing in the blood of virgins." Do we really think that if we are touched by youth, it somehow rubs off as an antidote to aging? You know I'm afraid to test that one out.

At age 40, you really shouldn't have to worry about your sexual prowess. Odds are, if you've been having satisfactory sexual activity, you'll continue to do so for a good long while yet. What is there to prove?

Your physical ability to have a good sex life, although ultimately bound to diminish with each decade, can, in a psychological way, be relatively unaffected as you get older. There are certain changes, but they don't mean that you can't stay in the game. If you are having problems, again look first to physical causes such as illness or alcohol abuse. To paraphrase Falstaff, alcohol increases the desire while playing hell with the performance.

Depression is another factor that can negatively affect men and women alike, decreasing interest in romance as well as sexual satisfaction. Here again, the issue is not sex; it's something else—depression, anxiety, grief from work, money, family problems, or loss of a lover.

Fear of Death and Other Inconveniences....Worry, Worry, Worry

The common belief is that as we age, we worry more about death. Studies show, however, that although thoughts about death are more frequent with age, a dread of death is actually less frequent as we approach the event. As it turns out, at midlife we are more likely to dread death than a nonagenarian who may be so much closer to the Grim Reaper. In fact, fear of death is much more common among the middle-aged than among the elderly.

Maybe this shouldn't come as a surprise. In middle age, we become aware of how much less time we have left compared to what has already passed. All too often, we are confronted by the death of a parent, a beloved mentor, a classmate, or a dear friend. This often forces on us an unwilling awareness of our own mortality. We begin to think more and more about the fact that we're mortal—rather a hard job for those of us who only a few years earlier thought we were unbreakable. Hey, wait a minute, that's not in my job description!

Anxiety about aging can lead to fear of death. We see this in untreated depressed individuals who are obsessed with thoughts of dying. Experts blame their depression on an internal chemical deficiency (serotonin) often associated with an early loss or separation or an unresolved painful conflict.

Fortunately, most of us have the resiliency to face even the end with equanimity. By and large, the terminally ill who are not clinically depressed show positive skills at accepting their fate, no matter how bleak that may be; and that is after they manage to get over all that denial and anger that Kubler-Ross would have us accept.

The Sandwich Generation

As I've mentioned before, a tremendous burden falls on the baby boom generation, who are forced to look after aging parents as well as their own families. This is in fact no different from many generations before us when it was more common to have multiple generations living under the same roof. But today life extends so much longer, and too often it can end not with a bang, but a whimper.

Owing to an increased life expectancy, today's middle-aged offspring are much more likely to have living parents and grandparents than did their parents or grandparents before them. Because of a decline in the current generation's fertility, parents may have less kin to call on for help than did their own parents when they begin to lose their health and power. When everyone gets counted, there are more living parents than living children—one big, but older, happy family.

So let's get back to the reason for bringing up these disparities in the size of the old and new generations. It ain't exactly a laugh riot being a baby boomer, sandwiched between equally demanding generations, struggling with careers, with nary a moment for ourselves to maintain health and fitness.

Most middle-aged adults have grown up in smaller families than a generation or two ago and have fewer siblings to share the psychological stress of taking care of their aging parents or in-laws. Furthermore, half of all married women are now in the work force. Women, at one time the mainstay of the family support system, now are unavailable. This increases the stress on male children, themselves aging, who must take on more of the responsibility of caring for aging parents—a duty we're rarely prepared for. The traditional nurturing role historically taken by women is now being assumed by more men, who at the same time are trying to deal with the problems of their children, their jobs, and money, along with what possibly can be the most threatening challenge, of all their own aging.

Caregiving is stressful. It often demands a restructuring of your own values, priorities, plans, and responsibilities. The time demand created by a beloved but deteriorating ill parent or parent-in-law can wreak havoc on a family relationship if you let it. He or she may actually become the object of resentment and, moving one step further, a cause of guilt from these feelings.

Once again, there's more than enough stress to go around.

Maintaining Sanity

As we age and acquire normal aches and pains, escalating concerns about changing physical, mental, and sexual prowess are easy to understand. Along with those concerns, we might begin to require a myriad of exotic medications just to stay even. We cease to take our health for granted. Indeed, it becomes more and more a focus of our existence.

The bottom line is that we must consider both genetic and environmental reasons for our responses to the stresses of midlife. The lucky ones among us maintain robust physical, mental, and sexual health nearly to the end of a long life. The unlucky ones age prematurely and may reach an early death or incapacity. Often there is very little justice to how we get placed in either category. I say to my children, "Who said life was fair?" They look at me quizically.s

And yet, lest you've missed the theme of this book, there are steps we can take to increase the odds in our favor—toward a complete life, physically, mentally, and spiritually. All this starts somewhere, and it doesn't arrive in the mail with the first Social Security check. The roots of these problems come earlier, as concerns for the future and especially in how you prepare yourselves for dealing with the aging process.

In other words, much of what you will become in later years starts now. Once you know where you stand, as young Hamlet counseled, you can "take arms against a sea of troubles, and by opposing, end them."

SUGGESTED READINGS

Cole, Thomas R. *The Oxford Book of Aging: Reflections on the Journey of Life.* Oxford, 1994. 419 pp.

Williams, Mark E. *Complete Guide to Aging and Health.* Harmony Books, 1995. 494 pp.

George Hovland

Aging With Amazing Grace

Over seven decades ago George Hovland made his entrance into the world. He was born in Duluth, Minnesota, to parents of Norwegian-German heritage. The neighborhood of his childhood would be the envy of any child, with a vast city park and ski hill practically at his back door. The natural beauty of the park combined with its unlimited opportunities for outdoor play was a perfect setting for George and his neighborhood friends to enjoy fun, yet subtly competitive, sports.

The era of George's youth was free of the technical toys that trap the youth of today indoors. Instead, George and the boys of his neighborhood spent endless carefree hours playing baseball and just about anything else this enthusiastic band of young athletes could think of. But it was winter that George yearned for most of all. For within the magic of winter lay the promise of a sport that would someday transform his life and create a passion that he would seek to share with others to this day. The sport he loved so passionately was skiing. And it would eventually take him from his beloved neighborhood park to the 1952 winter Olympics in Oslo, Norway, to compete in cross-country as a member of the U.S. Nordic Combine (jumping and cross-country) team.

Resting on past laurels is not George's style. The thrill of competition in all of the ski disciplines led him to win several four-event championships. He continued his Alpine racing career in the NASTAR (National Alpine Racing Program) where he won several National Championships, often beating racers less than half his age. George feels that all types of skiing should be a thing of grace and beauty; George's style makes skiing look effortless.

For many years, cross-country skiing has been George's main focus. As of this writing, he is planning to complete his 25th American Birkebeiner, where he has won his age group a number of times. This past season, he skied the 90-kilometer Swedish Vasaloppet, the race which he completed as the first non-European 45 years ago. His time, one hour slower than in 1952, was disappointing to him, but he still had great fun.

In the early 70s, as a thriving home designer and builder, George and his three children—Julie, George III, and Lee—would travel to various Minnesota and Wisconsin Alpine ski areas. He credits his children's enthusiasm and ability for motivating him to continue Alpine ski racing. Over the years, increasingly frustrated by the long drives, he was inspired to conceive of a local Alpine facility for the skiers of Duluth. Looking up at the beautiful Duluth hillside, he dreamed of a ski area right in the city's backyard. George's dream would become a reality when, on December

20, 1973, Duluthians celebrated the opening of Spirit Mountain. George reveled in the joy of bringing skiing closer to the youth of Duluth. It was only natural that it should happen and it's been fun for tens of thousands of skiers over the years.

In 1993, George and his wife Jane decided to take their love of cross-country skiing one step further. They created the Snowflake Nordic Center in Duluth, complete with a charming Scandinavian-style chalet, 15 kilometers of varied trails for tiny tots to Olympic hopefuls, and a 6-kilometer lighted trail for busy Duluthians.

When George semi-retired from his contracting business, he thought that it would afford him more time for skiing. Unfortunately, George states with conviction from his experience that if you want to ski a lot, don't own and operate a cross-country ski center. His enthusiasm for skiing is still high, and he looks forward to each new day, to the beauty of winter, to the thrills of skiing, and to the enjoyment of fellow skiers. George often quotes his 91-year-old Norwegian friend Pete Fosseide, who said many years ago, "Skiing is a very healthy sport."

To this day, you would be hard-pressed to convince anyone that George is 71. In fact, when he attempts to take advantage of senior citizen discounts he is required to show his driver's license. Even then they don't believe him! George Hovland is proof positive that living a healthy, active lifestyle is the key to aging with amazing grace.

Chapter 6

Aging Can Be Good
■ Stretch, Aerobicize, and Pump Iron

A strong body makes the mind strong. —Thomas Jefferson

The male is an animal that is genetically, environmentally, and perhaps even spiritually conditioned to exert himself physically for his livelihood. Yet it still doesn't take much for this same animal to get out of shape physically and mentally. And when our human male starts letting himself go, there can be many consequences...most bad. He starts to take losses in terms of increased disability, not to mention susceptibility to illness. He also begins to feel bad about himself. Being out of shape causes him stress and internal turmoil that, like a domino effect, contribute to further physical problems. And as he lets his body slide, maybe, if he's lucky, he realizes somewhere deep inside that letting himself go is fundamentally wrong.

Midlife is especially a critical time for us males (grunt, grunt!). We have long ago left behind those years when we thought we could do just about anything we wanted with our bodies and survive unscathed. We've started to feel our years. We now suffer aches and pains after exercising. We may have begun to notice a decline in our physical performance. So that we may also begin to look ahead to the rest of our life possibly with dread, thus producing even more stress.

More damned reality: "Muscle strength usually decreases 20 percent between the ages of 22 and 65; bone mass and, worse yet, flexibility, also decreases with age" (American College of Sports Medicine *Syllabus,* 1996).

So what else is new that we didn't know already?

Now for some happy news: Midlife can also be a time of opportunity. We still retain enough of our physical strength and stamina that if we take action now, we can preserve our performance, restore our sense of well-being, and still prepare ourselves physically and mentally for some great years.

Do We Really Have to Fall Apart? Here's How Not To

It all comes down to culture—the environment, society, and era in which we live. The fact is that in North America, as well as other so-called advanced Western societies, we can live in a culture of inactivity. We've heard a lot of reasons for this phenomenon: the movement of work from outside to inside, from body to brain, from physical activity to physical passivity. Commensurately, our time for recreation and leisure has increased, leading to more time sitting than standing or moving about. The human culture has traditionally viewed leisure as a passive activity—a break from an often backbreaking day of work. Ironically, the day's toils are, for most men, now largely physically passive, and leisure time can provide the only opportunity for physical activity.

American males come from a hodgepodge of sources. A few arrived on these shores wealthy; others came as slaves. Still others came for work in our fields and factories, building our railroads and cities. Many are the descendants of the dregs of Europe, sprung from a motley collection of convicts or near-convicts, drifters, religious fanatics, impoverished farmers and laborers, or assorted groups of oppressed rebels. The British, for example, before they began sending their political prisoners to Australia, used to send them to America.

The common denominator was often work. We arrived in America to earn a living by the sweat of our brow. Immigrants who have followed from other cultures—such as Asian and Latin American in particular—are no exception. Our beginnings were decidedly blue-collar. Most Americans have had to earn their livings from plain hard work. Yet (as now), the workplace has tended to be harshly exploitative.

In this setting, any notion of fun became synonymous with total inactivity. Movement is duty. Sitting around motionless with the wife and kids on Sunday in front of "the tube" can be the cherished ideal of the good life. The same applies to that once famous tradition, the Sunday family drive to the country after church and the big Sunday meal. As the old saw goes, "Anybody who has to exercise after a busy day on the farm hasn't worked hard enough." You've come a long way, baby, with air-conditioned tractors and CDs du jour.

This ethos can go mighty deep. Look at a simple device such as self-propelled lawnmower. We go out and spend hundreds of dollars to buy a machine that drinks gas and belches out carbon monoxide and other pollutants, all the while denying us the same exercise that we pay hundreds of dollars a year for at a fitness club. Ditto for a leaf blower, which accomplishes a function that can be done just as well (and probably nearly as quickly) with a $10 rake. My recommendation is (1) don't buy a leaf blower, (2) buy a $10 rake, (3) help prevent air pollution, and (4) earn calorie credits for your dinner by raking and collecting your leaves.

Exercise-O-Phobia

Starting an exercise program can be like starting to write a book—that impending task can seem overwhelmingly daunting. Thus, like a writer with writer's block, the truly inveterate couch potato can experience "exercise block" with the best of them. In both cases, such laziness can lead to a nasty cycle of militant inactivity.

Observe children: Once, they rarely stopped moving from morning till night. These days, though, television, Nintendo, automation, urbanization, and the automobile have turned many kids into brainwashed little pairs of staring eyes. And we too contribute. What kind of example are male adults giving when we are guilty of the same sin? How many times have I seen parents haul their wee ones off to soccer or ice-skating or little league only to sit passively on the sideline till the event is over?

Genetic studies give strong credence to the adage "fat parents make fat children." Behavioral example does the same.

Establishing a Fitness Habit Is Not Easy

You can use a variety of incentives to psych yourself up for getting into shape, ranging from the personal to the scientific. It doesn't hurt to repeat to yourself every night before you go to bed and every morning as you stare at your paunch in the mirror statements such as:

"I need to get that gut off before we go to the beach this summer."

"Being in shape makes me feel good, and I look better too."

"Regular strength training, even when I'm older, can increase muscle strength, bone mass, and flexibility."

"I can reverse, or at best slow, the seemingly inevitable deterioration caused by the aging process."

"Being in shape makes me a better father/worker/boss/husband/lover."

Having a positive attitude can be a start, but the couch potato cum exercise monster still has a ways to go.

First, the Bad News

As men, we've been conditioned to think we can ignore our bodies. We've come to believe it's not macho to admit disability or discomfort, something about "big boys don't cry." We just expect our bodies to work, and we're especially proud if we can keep some level of fitness while hardly seeming to try. Working against us here is the fact that having to do anything to remain fit is subconsciously seen not as something real men have to do. I'm a real man and have to consistently work very hard to keep the wolf from the door.

Habits built over half a lifetime can be hard to break. The greatest hurdle for anyone over 40 is making the decision to stay fit or, even harder, restarting a physical conditioning program. It is just so much easier to wake up, brew some coffee, smear a bagel with cream cheese, and then hunker down to the morning paper. I'm at a point in life where I do the bagel first and run later when the sun is at full mast. The over-40 guy who wants to initiate an exercise regimen frequently may have to overcome built-in cultural inhibitors—in other words, he has to *really want* to get his physical life in order and work exercise into his hectic schedule. Priorities, priorities, priorities. At the very core of this struggle is the place exercise must occupy on our priority list. It always seems so easily expendable when "duty" calls. Chalk this way of thinking up to the age-old (and aforementioned) American work ethic—business first. Run a little behind on a deadline, and so will the trip to the health club. "I'm late, I'm late for a very important date...."

This approach to life may carry you through your thirties—those years critical to establishing a financial base—but now, as you enter your forties, the ever-increasing aches and pains coupled with diminishing flexibility and stamina force you into a tough decision: Are you going to keep exercise and wellness down a few pegs on the list? What are you going to do with the truth that life without fitness and health may not work any longer?

The worst mistake is to believe that it's too late to begin or that you're too over-the-hill to recover any aspect of your now-faded youth. Or is it the fear of the pain you know may accompany getting back into shape?

Whatever the mental block is, the solution is to say, "what the hell?" Draw on that age-old male trait of simply barging ahead with little rhyme or reason—you know, the one that used to get us in trouble during our impetuous youth? Put it to good use now: Genetically, that might be what it's there for. So here's the plan: Exercise first, work later.

Now for the Good News

It's never too late to start. And beginning an exercise program doesn't have to mean killing yourself in a gym. It means simply starting to move, beating the ennui. Here are a few pertinent truths to get you going:

1. Escalators and elevators don't do anything to help your heart. So take the stairs.
2. The longer you play with your kids, the longer you will be able to play with your grandkids.
3. Don't park close to the mall entrance. Cars parked close to the mall are more likely to be dented. So park far and walk.
4. Biking to work prevents pollution and builds your quads.
5. A twice-daily tour around the block can help prevent neighborhood crime.

6. A walk with your wife can prevent divorce; a walk with your kids can prevent juvenile delinquency and maybe even teenage pregnancy.

7. Sweat smells sexy. (Really?)

8. If you walk to the supermarket, you can carry less home and therefore may buy less, make more trips, get more exercise, and maybe even lose some weight.

9. Pushing a lawnmower, raking leaves, and shoveling snow are all good for the environment—both yours and everyone else's.

10. Prolonged television watching creates both physical and mental flab.

The moral of the story: Become a doer, not a watcher. A participant, not a spectator. A facilitator, not a couch potater.

Once you've come this far, now it's time to...**THINK MOSH**

Motivation is the key

Remember, it's **O**K to exercise

Schedule your workouts

If it **H**urts, stop!

Motivation Is the Key

It helps to have a vision of some kind—a focus to keep up your motivation. Come up with a picture of what you want to look like, feel like, or be like. Maybe conjure up a sports or movie hero. Nolan Ryan was throwing fireballs well into his forties while guys half his age had long ago dreamed up excuses for quitting baseball. Satchel Paige was serving up curveballs to major-league batters in his sixties.

One method of priming your motivation is to relate your newfound commitment to a part of you that was once active. Think of it as going back to gym again, when you got to turn your back on your math teacher and have fun at school for a change. Despite eternally sweaty gym clothes and cold locker rooms, gym was a welcome break for most of us. Remember this wonderful part of your life when you could really be *male?*

It's probably especially helpful to focus on what you weighed at the end of high school. Maybe the most realistic notion is getting yourself within 10 to 20 pounds of what you weighed in those golden years.

Conjure up all the *positive* reasons for working out. For example:

■ Exercise increases the speed at which food is metabolized. It sets your engine idle a bit higher. You can eat more yet wear it less.

■ Exercise activates your body during awake periods, and then tuckers you out for a deeper, more consistent sleep.

■ Exercise helps your body avoid the ravages of chronic health problems such as heart disease, arthritis, diabetes, and osteoporosis.

- Exercise builds self-confidence, improves the ability to relax, and fights depression. It makes you feel better about yourself. You're doing something instead of veging out in front of the TV or relying on one too many cocktails to help you settle down after the day.
- Exercise makes you look better. And when you look better, people tend to hold you in higher esteem.
- Exercising can make you a more exciting lover. Hey, what are women attracted to? Sensitivity and caring are at the top of the list, but also up there are self-confidence and good looks. 'Nuff said.

Remember, It's OK to Exercise

One major roadblock to exercise is that some people—including a few unenlightened wives and employers—believe that exercise is self-indulgent or narcissistic, or that your time is better spent doing something else.

You have a right to exercise. Fortunately, most wives and girlfriends realize that allowing you time to exercise is better in the long run for them, too. Many want to participate actively *with* you. And more employers are allowing schedule flexibility and even providing facilities for employees to work out. Many large corporations—Microsoft is a good example—promote intramural sports teams, realizing that this builds company spirit and thus a more productive workplace. Of course, they can also lower health insurance premiums by having healthier employees.

Exercise can be the chance to turn off pesky negative programs that often clutter up the brain. Remember recess in grade school? It was a good idea then. It's a good idea now.

Schedule Your Workouts

The sad reality that strikes almost everyone about to exercise after a hard day at the office is that it takes a lot of perseverance, self-control, and self-focus just to hit the gym. For starters, you may be hungry, and dinner begins to sound mighty inviting. Sure, there are those who work out after dinner, but if that were you, you probably wouldn't be reading this.

One secret I've discovered is simply to put exercise on your schedule just like any other family or work event and stick to it. Of course, discuss this decision with your family and even your boss first. Hopefully, they'll realize that they'll be primary beneficiaries of "the new you"—unless they prefer you as a flabby, stressed-out individual subject to early disability or even death.

If It Hurts, Stop!

Your body is smarter than you think—perhaps even a lot smarter than you are. It knows it needs exercise, even if you don't, and also knows when you might be overdoing it. So listen to your body. If you start hurting, you're doing too much, going too fast, keeping at it too long, or lifting too much. Perhaps you aren't properly warmed up—more on that later. In any case, your exercise should remain within an acceptable, intelligent comfort zone.

There's a rule of thumb that if you're running strictly for training, not racing, you should be able to carry on a conversation while you run. If you find you can't, you're probably going anaerobic—your body is going into the red—and lactate is building up in your muscles. Later, if you really get into exercise and do achieve a high level of fitness, there will be times that your workouts tend to ignore such limitations. But when you're just getting started, this is a good principle to follow.

Remember, too, that just because you're male doesn't mean you're in competition. You're not out to beat or even keep up with the other runners, male or female, especially if they've been at it longer than you. There's no such thing as going too slow, and no dishonor will ever come from starting out in low gear. Accept "going slow" at first and try your hand at walking, hiking, biking, or swimming. At each sport, you can find your own level, your own comfort zone, both physically and mentally. In short, if you can't escape your type A behavior, at least leave it at the office.

WHEN NOT TO EXERCISE

There are times when you **shouldn't** exercise. When any one or more of the following conditions exist, it may be time to take a rest.

You have an unexpected physical symptom such as chest pain, pain in joints, or light-headedness, especially if it begins or is made worse with exercise.

You are in a location where you are not used to the climate—for example, high altitude or extreme heat, humidity, or cold.

You are visiting a city that has a high smog level—e.g., Mexico City, Los Angeles, Denver, Washington, New York.

You've just had a heavy meal.

You partied too hard the night before. (You're hungover.)

You've consumed too much soda, tea, or coffee, especially if you are unaccustomed to their effect.

You are taking certain drugs (antidepressants such as imipramine, for instance) that can elevate your baseline heart rate.

You are using strong decongestants or antihistamines, which cause dehydration.

You're suffering from prolonged fatigue (over 24 hours).

You're having trouble sleeping (insomnia), and exercise only makes it worse.

You have a rapid resting (awakening) heartbeat.

A Few Caveats

You can't just go from being a ripe couch potato to Mr. Fitness, even if you have made the mental commitment. As in any major lifestyle change, there has to be a gradual process. Also, once you've begun the journey, you need to be aware continuously of your body's needs.

Get Tested First

Very important: Before you begin an exercise regimen, schedule a thorough medical history and physical exam with your health care practitioner (HCP). Announce your intentions and see what reaction you get. Your MD (doctor), PA (physician's assistant), or NP (nurse practitioner) will doubtless encourage you but may pale at the thought of letting you drag your body through a tough physical regimen. You may have to take charge and let her know the sincerity of your intentions. Make sure you receive a complete laboratory study, including
- blood count
- fasting chemistry profile for cholesterol
- triglyceride, liver, and renal function tests
- EKG (electrocardiogram)
- urinalysis

Create a partnership with your HCP. There is much he or she can do to promote "the new you." For example, your HCP may suggest appropriate heart rates to shoot for during exercise. If you show a high cholesterol, your HCP might suggest dietary and weight intervention in addition to upping the throttle on exercise. Be aware, however, that many "old-school" physicians may be somewhat unenlightened on the subject of nutrition. They tend to think intervention rather than prevention. Be prepared to chart your own course, which is why there is a chapter later in this book to help you with this challenge. Also consider scheduling routine hearing and vision evaluations; they're just as important for you as they are for any fourth grader.

Be Aware of Your Body

Letting someone else check you over is a great start, but you are your own best health monitor. At the tender age of 40 and above, you should be keeping a watchful eye on the following:

1. Your upper GI tract. The food tube. Look for pain in swallowing or if you experience any other discomfort when you eat. And if you find yourself vomiting blood, get thee to medical care posthaste!

2. Your lower GI tract. Blood in your stool might indicate anything from hemorrhoids (generally not a big deal) to colon or rectal cancer (a really big deal).

3. Your urine. Does it smell sweet? Are you urinating a lot? Are you constantly thirsty? Any of these symptoms might indicate high blood sugar. Be aware of your family history. Type 2 (adult-onset) diabetes is hereditary.

4. Your blood (part 1). If any of the above symptoms apply, get your blood checked.

5. Your blood (part 2). Low serum iron and hemoglobin levels may indicate anemia either from internal bleeding or other illness such as infection, tissue disorder, or even cancer. This can be checked any time you get your blood tested. But because you're not going in for a physical more than once a year, here's how to get it done more often: You can kill two birds with one stone by donating blood regularly. Usually you can give every 56 days. As part of the predonation testing, the Red Cross (or whomever you are donating to) will check your hemoglobin level.

Note carefully: Smoking can cause high iron and hemoglobin levels in the blood by increasing carbon monoxide (CO) and decreasing oxygen saturation (O_2) in the blood.

6. Your skin. Do you have any new moles or an old one that's suddenly changing color, size, or shape? If it's showing any sign of change, see your HCP as soon as possible. You'll want the mole excised, punch biopsied, or widely dissected.

Other Reminders: Basic Health Stuff

Beginning an exercise program and monitoring your health are two great steps toward becoming one with an active lifestyle. A third, which easily goes hand in hand, is taking better care of yourself. For example:

1. Be aware of sun exposure. Being outside in the sun is good, especially during those rough winter months. The sun serves up vitamin D, a necessary catalyst for using calcium for healthy bones and other body functions. But during the summer, be careful not to get too much sun, which can be a primary cause of skin cancer. Stay out of the direct midday sun as much as possible, especially without 35+ sunscreen. If you must get sun, expose the bod before 11:00 or after 2:00, and even then use 15+ sunscreen, adding heavier stuff on the nose, ears, neck, and shoulders. Remember, water washes off sunscreen (despite manufacturer claims of being waterproof), and water also reflects sun, in effect giving you a concentrated exposure. Also be aware that the higher you are in altitude, the less atmosphere there is to protect you from the sun's more harmful rays. Aspen may be cooler than Death Valley, but you can get burned just as easily. One more bit of advice: Buy a hat and wear it!

2. Consume plenty of fluid… like plain old water. So you don't like the stuff that comes out of the tap? Buy bottled water; it comes in many flavors.

3. Limit fat intake, especially saturated fats, particularly animal fats. Some fat is good and necessary. In fact, I advocate the judicious use of olive oil. So-called Mediterranean diets—which use almost exclusively olive oil and feature copious amounts of fresh fruits and vegetables, not to mention wine—seem to promote greater longevity. And there is laboratory evidence to back up the positive attributes of olive oil.

4. Get periodic medical checkups. Once every two years is usually right.

5. Drink alcoholic beverages in moderation. We all have a different tolerance level—don't try to keep up with your neighbor who plays offensive guard for the San Francisco 49ers. I favor good wine and beer over hard liquor because wine and beer go better with meals. And there are certain schools of thought that advocate a glass or two of red wine a day for better health. I'm not arguing, but I'm not going to overdo it either.

6. You can quit smoking! This is the big one. As you age, your lungs usually become less efficient. If you smoke, such changes become even worse. People who smoke tend to (1) have less healthy lives and (2) die earlier. Period. Sure, we've all heard about the octogenarian who's been smoking a pack a day from the time he was 17. But trust me, this is rare. That's why you hear about it. Remember, if it's news, it's not commonplace.

What doesn't stick out in memory are the examples of folks who lived for year after year tethered to an oxygen tank or slowly withered away from lung cancer in a nursing home. Believe me, I've seen it: Life is not much fun when you're gasping for each breath.

So if you want a long and physically happy life, you must quit smoking. Besides, there's a day coming when smokers may be denied more than just seats in restaurants. Smoking may constitute an automatic disqualification for preferred rates on health insurance… or any health insurance at all.

If you've been a smoker for any length of time and you're over 40, yearly screening chest X rays become imperative. So you want to quit today? Here's the good news: Anyone who has been smoke-free for more than 10 years is no more likely to get cancer than someone who has never smoked—certainly an inducement to quit early.

Here's where I get on my soapbox.

We've been conditioned as a society to take a live-and-let-live approach to smoking. That's wrong. It amounts to live-and-let-die. Smoking costs us billions of dollars each year in health care costs, pain and suffering, lost work, and lost loved ones. This loss comes directly out of our pockets and our lives.

How do you quit?

There are as many methods as there are smokers who want to quit. Some simply go cold turkey. Some taper off. Many remove all vestiges of smoking from their houses—cigarettes, ashtrays, matches and lighters, even spouses who aren't ready to kick the habit. They refuse to go to bars where smoking goes hand in hand with drinking. They chew on fresh vegetables such as carrots and celery for that oral fix. They tell themselves over and over how strong they are to undergo this addiction withdrawal. And you know something? They are!

There are other methods: Various nicotine gums or one of several nicotine patches, either alone or in conjunction with a smoke cessation program, can mean the end of your mean habit. Nicotine replacement is considered generally safe except in the worst of heart conditions or if you decide to smoke while on the patch. Certain enlightened insurance companies will reimburse you for using the patch. Some require completion of a year's smoking cessation before they do so. How's that for intimidation, I mean motivation?

There is also a new smoking cessation medication called Z-Bann, which is actually long Wellbutrin tablets (150mg) taken twice a day that rely on their anticompulsive properties. In actuality, Wellbutrin is another of the serotonin reuptake inhibitors. Although studies support the efficacy of Wellbutrin, this practitioner has yet to confirm the success stories. The drug, like the other seratonin reuptake inhibitors, tends to be a bit pricey.

What if you don't smoke, but someone you care about does? That's tough, because smokers don't want to be told to give it up. There are techniques that work for alcoholics that can also help smokers kick their habit. On the positive side, you can offer to pay for a smoke-enders program or nicotine patches. You can offer a reward such as a cruise, car, or 24-carat diamond ring—that is, bribery. Don't be afraid to take a strong stand about stopping smoking. After all, if you love someone, you want them to be healthy and ultimately happy.

The Main Event

Now that you've made your commitment and become more aware of what's better for the body, it's time to get down and do it! There are three basic elements of the exercise routine—stretching, aerobics, and strength training.

Don't Forget to Stretch

For some reason, stretching has never been a "guy thing." There's something perceived as kind of feminine about taking 30 minutes out of the day or away from your sport of choice just to lie on the floor and focus on special taut parts of your body.

This has to change if you want a long and happy, pain-free, fit life. Stretching has to become an integral part of any physical conditioning program so that even if you choose to remain a couch potato, you'll be able to get up painlessly from that couch when you need to go to the fridge for beers and munchies.

If you do choose to exercise—of course, that's the goal—stretching helps prevent injuries. It enables you to work out harder, longer, and without discomfort both during and after exercising. It can help you maintain maximum range of motion in your joints. The benefits of stretching are progressive. The more you stretch, the easier it becomes, and the more flexible your body will be. In the next chapter, I'll give you some suggestions on how to get maximum effect from a few simple stretches. Don't worry, there will be nothing here akin to Richard Simmons.

Go for the Aerobics

As we discussed earlier, all of our muscles are subject to the rigors of aging. The heart, very much a muscle, is no exception, especially in men. Similarly, like every other muscle in your body, the heart also responds to conditioning. The weight it gains as you age is often deposited as less functional fibrous tissue; you must do everything possible to counteract the natural tendency for your heart muscles (the working part of your heart) to shrink and lose myocardial fibrils and become replaced by less functional fibrous tissue. The goal with age is to nurture not only a big heart but a strong heart.

As we age, our heart rate decreases. There's no getting around it. Yet as you grow older, you can compensate—and even overcompensate—just by increasing the amount of blood the heart pumps per stroke (called cardiac output). Aerobic conditioning accomplishes this by making the heart more efficient. Aerobic conditioning also strengthens the muscles in your chest wall and may be the one way to counteract the inexorable decrease in lung performance.

Don't Neglect Strength Training

In the recent push toward aerobic exercise, old-fashioned exercise for strength may have been forgotten for a while. It shouldn't be. The American College of Sports Medicine (ACSM) now recommends that we participate in strength-training exercises at least twice a week. There's good reason for this. As you mature, you tend to lose muscle mass only to replace it with fat, which is much lighter and less useful (except to help you float better). One way you can avoid losing muscle is simply to look for easy, natural ways to incorporate strength workouts into your lifestyle. I mentioned earlier pushing a manual lawnmower, raking leaves, and shoveling snow; eschewing escalators and elevators for stairs; walking or riding a bike instead of driving your car. Even washing windows can have beneficial effects on muscles. And you don't even have to head to the gym to use Nautilus.

In the gym, there's no need to be macho man and lift weights with the youngsters. You can if you want, and in fact I know men in their fifties who've successfully transitioned from a relatively sedentary, heavy drinking, heavy smoking lifestyle to one of pumping iron with the big boys. If weight lifting isn't your bag, try the various muscle-toning machines that are designed to provide maximum steady resistance to a wide range of muscles. You won't put on bulk using these machines, but you will work your muscles to their maximum efficiency. (And you'll look better, too!)

To Sum Up

Don't expect fitness or its habit just to happen. Plan to ease into the process slowly. The biggest mistake for the born-again-to-fitness 40 year old is the danger of overdoing it. The rejuvenated 40-year-old wanna-be weekend athlete who overdoes the squats may instead only learn to equate pain with his newly chosen life of exercise and what should be "fun."

Living healthy makes you feel better, but you may not live longer. Exercising three times a week to a sweat, for about 30 to 40 minutes, can help preserve what you've got left. Subsequently maintaining ideal body weight can decrease hypertension and help prevent the onset of Type 2 diabetes.

Make exercise a part of your life. It may seem strange at first—even a bit self-indulgent—but it will have increasing benefits for you, your life, and your loved ones.

Just think: It's recess once again, boys.

SUGGESTED READING

Garbammer, John. *Strength Training.* Sports Illustrated Book, 1994. 204 pp.

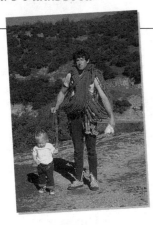

Rick Sylvester

Stuntman

When I met Rick on the balcony of the Telemark Lodge the day before the North American Birkebeiner, the largest cross-country ski race in North America, I was hard-pressed to believe that this smallish, curly-haired guy had actually been a James Bond stuntman. At that time I must have been the only over-40 male in America who had not seen the famous sequence in *The Spy Who Loved Me* where Agent 007 skis recklessly down a Baffin Island slope, shoots off a sheer ledge, kicks off his skis, and floats easily to safety under a billowy Union Jack parachute. Of course, that was not really James Bond—or rather Roger Moore, who was playing Bond at the time. It was Rick.

Rick went on to double for James Bond in *For Your Eyes Only.* In one stunt for Roger, Rick did a complete free fall from a climbing rope on the Greek island of Meteora.

Despite his small size, Rick has always been an athlete. At 130 pounds, he was an NCAA champion wrestler at the University of California at Berkeley back in the sixties. And sport was why Sylvester, independently comfortable from his father's successful Southern California developments, moved to the Lake Tahoe–Squaw Valley area in the mid-1970s because of its opportunities for running and climbing during the warmer months, and skiing during the winter. He still lives there today with his two children and wife Betsy.

Being a James Bond stuntman is quite a life, so the question "What are you going to do for an encore?" has hit Rick hard. Like all guys reaching their fifties, trying to keep up with the pack is getting tougher and tougher. One problem is motivation. "Somehow, after all these years," he says, "I need more variety, new trails and runs, different climbs." But more tough to swallow is just plain getting older.

In the past, Rick has been a year-round runner, switching to his true passion, climbing, in the warmer months. This is a guy who used to cross-country ski the 230-mile John Muir High Ridge Trail. This is a guy who took up cross-country ski racing in his forties and placed in major races nationally—especially in the 50K events. This is a guy who used to enter many of Europe's major ski marathons regularly. Yet today he understandably gets frustrated when he can't keep up with the younger guys the way he once did.

Rick, however, has adapted. If three workouts a day leave him with no energy, he switches from competitive skiing to touring, and from running to roller skiing to ease the stress on the legs, knees, and ankles.

Like anyone who pushes hard day after day, he has brought his body to the edge, both literally and figuratively. At one point, a complete lack of energy led him to a cardiologist in nearby Reno. All tests were negative, except that his cholesterol was hovering around an ominous 270. Diet failed to make this number budge, but medication brought him down to a respectable 170. In the process, he and his family dropped all red meat. This was after a complete cardiovascular evaluation.

Despite bouts with low white cell counts and learning that some of his stunts had left more damage than he previously thought, Rick maintains a clear perspective on growing old. Although going out and exercising is more difficult than it used to be, he nevertheless keeps at it. In his mid-fifties, he's still a spry 140 pounds. And he takes pride in seeing himself featured in *Hollywood's Greatest Stunts.* Slowed down, yes. No longer 35, yes. Still staying active, absolutely. But skiing off sheer cliffs he's stopped. Intelligently, he's leaving that for the younger crowd.

Chapter 7

Recent History and Theory of Exercising

■ What, Why, and How

Middle age is when your age begins to show around the middle.

Bob Hope

Once you've decided to get into shape—or that you're going to retain the shape you're already in, assuming it's pretty good—the object is to design a fitness program that you can stick with, one that will provide maximum benefit for the time you spend at it. Your regimen should be enjoyable and give you benefits for your mind as well as your body—that old Greek ideal again.

Here's how you do it.

Exercises for Strength

Strength training can do a number of things for you that tend to get forgotten in this age of aerobic mania. Ubiquitous health clubs everywhere promote cardiovascular fitness that, without question, has been the watchword to the exercise set. Yet strength training, too, especially now and at later stages of your life, must not be forgotten. There are good reasons for this.

First, strength training, as much as stretching for your warm-up and especially your cooldown, is a critical element in preventing injury. By conditioning opposing muscle groups (e.g., quads versus hamstrings, triceps versus biceps), you can strengthen the maximal number of joints and tendons connected to those muscles. One way that well-conditioned muscles can protect joints is simply by preventing hyperextension. Hyperextension is what makes the delicate (and hard-to-heal) tendons and ligaments crack like dry spaghetti. For example, if you have weak knees, you should strengthen opposing leg muscles around the knee: quadriceps versus hamstrings, calf muscles opposing the muscles at the front of your legs (anterior tibialis) and the tendons around this crucial joint.

Have you ever had a shoulder separation? If so, I don't need to tell you the wisdom of strengthening your arm, back, shoulders, or any of the rotator cuff muscles above or behind your shoulder. A systematic muscle-strengthening program can make the potentially unstable shoulder joint stronger.

Second, strength training can also increase your performance by making you more powerful. By carefully strengthening neglected muscles, you can protect muscle groups that are not necessarily sports specific for you.

Third, there's vanity. Those in the bodybuilding trade jokingly refer to the process of strengthening your biceps as producing "curls for the girls," because your biceps may have little significance athletically other than to enhance your physique and make you look better on a New Jersey beach. So Bruce Springsteen really does have a reason for lifting.

Strength training can do more than protect your joints. Any injury to a large muscle group, such as your hamstrings or quadriceps, can often be overcome and very likely repaired by high-repetition, low-weight exercises specific to the injured muscles and those around them. This seems like such a novel, almost contradictory concept—that frequent contraction and then relaxation of an injured muscle can actually work to repair it. By doing low-weight, high-repetition exercises, you can actually strengthen those muscle fibrils that are still intact and not injured. Meanwhile, you can improve blood supply and oxygenation to injured muscles, thus helping to repair them.

Muscular strength is the amount of force a muscle can exert against any given resistance. There are plenty of ways to increase muscular strength. You can strengthen a muscle by overloading it—that is, by forcing it to work at greater loads than usual. Or you can do lighter work at increased repetitions. Some muscle groups respond better to one technique than to the other, and each method is good for specific types of muscular conditioning. Your arms and legs, for example, respond well to overload training; your abdominals and pectorals respond best to low-resistance, high-repetition exercise.

If you're looking for the most rapid gains in strength, you can exercise a particular muscle group at 80 to 100 percent of maximum. However, because there's a lot to be said for going "slow and low" to help avoid unnecessary injuries, remember that you can still develop strength with exercise intensities of 60 percent of maximum. Using this approach lessens your possibility of "bulking up."

Muscular endurance, on the other hand, requires exercising muscle groups at lower intensities and higher repetitions to the point of fatigue. As they say, "no pain, no gain."

An important concept is the "overload" principle, which states that the amount of weight must increase as the muscle gets stronger—the "progressive resistance" theory. This is the basis for weight training programs and why lifters so frequently boast about the amount of weight they can lift, press, or squat. "Gosh, I can bench press my grandmother plus 150 pounds. How much can you lift?" It's their measure of how well they're doing. Weight training is also extremely versatile. Done properly (ideally with expert supervision), there is a great deal of specificity—of your contraction, your training intensity, your training velocity, and the pattern of your movements. Let's call it an art form.

The methods of developing muscular strength are categorized according to types of muscular contraction regimens: isometric, isotonic (concentric or eccentric), and isokinetic training.

Isometric contraction is when you hold your muscle in a fixed position for a length of time while increasing tension on it. Its value to you athletically is limited because you gain more if a muscle is in motion. Isometric exercises were a technique many of us employed in training during the sixties. They can still be very useful because many of these exercises can be done virtually anywhere and without equipment. Admittedly, during isotonics you look as if you're performing tai chi.

Isotonic training techniques rely on a three-step program using 5 to 10 repetitions, three to five days a week. They consist of both *concentric* and *eccentric* contractions performed against either a constant or a variable resistance. The idea is to work the muscle to increasing fatigue by the time you get to the last repetition. In concentric contraction, the muscle shortens while overcoming a constant resistance; in eccentric contraction, a muscle lengthens under a constant resistance. Most training programs employ the concentric version.

In this jet-age society of ours where time is money, fitness buffs often prefer the *isokinetic* method of strengthening muscles. This way incorporates specialized (and often expensive) equipment, allowing muscles to develop maximal tension while shortening at a constant speed throughout a complete range of motion. With this approach, there are definite sport-specific advantages to the Nautilus or Cybex machines, which can simulate exercise movements in a carefully controlled setting. Researchers note that the isokinetic method has an advantage over isotonic and isometric techniques because of the opportunity to develop maximal force through a full range of motion, and because it allows an individual to develop strength at variable speeds.

According to Bob Moffatt, PhD, Professor in the Department of Movement and Physical Education at Florida State, the principles for developing strength and endurance in isokinetic training are the same as for isotonic strength training. Three sets are performed for each exercise, with 5 to 10 repetitions per set, three to five days a week, at speeds ranging from 24 to 180 degrees per second (if you are in the market for building strength).

Another technique is circuit training—that is, moving from exercise to exercise in a set routine that is then repeated. This training method can be used to develop increased muscular strength with low-repetition, high-resistance exercises while boosting aerobic capacity. Keep moving around the circuit, nonstop, and watch your heart rate soar. Generally, do 6 to 10 stations per circuit, repeating them two to three times per session. Perform as many repetitions as possible at 40 to 60 percent of maximal strength, with 15 to 30 seconds of rest between each exercise station.

There's no need to invest heavily in equipment. You'll find that you can do some very simple resistance exercises just using the weight of your own body, ranging from push-ups to pull-ups, stair climbing, and some easily constructed dynamic machines such as a roller or sliding board (developed in former East Germany) that can strengthen upper or lower body muscles easily and cheaply. The overall goal should be to make exercise fun, convenient, and easy—a good habit that you can take with you wherever you go. Exercising can be a way to feel stronger, reduce stress, or just feel better about yourself, especially as you perform your exercises with ever increasing finesse.

There are several muscle groups that need attention on a consistent basis:

- thigh
- calf
- back
- wrist, hand, forearm
- abdomen
- foot and ankle
- shoulder
- chest
- upper arm
- lower back and bottom (gluteus maximus, or "gluts")

Most of these represent muscles that oppose each other. It is important that you design a strength-training program that ensures a proper balance between primary and opposing muscles, such as the hamstring versus the quads and the stomach versus the back. If you neglect them, you have a greater chance of injuring a weaker opposing muscle.

A good example of opposing muscles is the quadriceps-hamstring duo—the muscles in the front and in the back of the thigh, respectively. The rule of thumb is that the weight you can lift with a primary muscle group, such as your quads (on a Nautilus machine, for example), should be about twice what you can lift with the opposing group such as your hamstrings. So if you can lift 200 pounds with your quads, you should be able to "curl" 100 pounds with your hamstrings. For most of us, such detailed measurement of the weights is not essential. But if you exercise one muscle of a pair, you damned well better exercise the other. Doing this, you can look forward to an uninjured fitness program.

In *Personalized Weight Training for Fitness and Athletics From Theory to Practice,* Frederick C. Hatfield, PhD, of *Muscle & Fitness* magazine, and March Krotee, PhD, of the Department of Kinesiology and Leisure Studies at the University of Minnesota, give a handy overview that has helped me understand how to get started with my own personalized strength-training program.

Muscle Types

Generally, it's helpful to know that there are two types of muscle fibers. The first is a red muscle, or slow-twitch (Type I) fiber, and the second is a white muscle, or fast-twitch (Type II) fiber. Slow-twitch muscles have greater oxidative capacity (i.e., they use more oxygen) and greater endurance (aerobic) capacity. They are chock full of mitochondria (the little energy units in all muscle), are highly capillarized (i.e., have lots of blood supply), and hold plenty of energy chemicals. They comprise the dark meat on the legs and wings of the fowl.

White, or fast-twitch, fibers are best suited for bursts of speed. Unlike dark fibers, white fibers vary considerably in respect to their endurance capacity. With variable oxidative capacity, fast-twitch fibers depend on high-energy compounds that power skeletal muscle contraction and form phosphates, rather than on enhancing the size and number of energy units and increasing capillarization around muscle fibers (the secret to fitness of slow-twitch muscles). Endurance exercise nonetheless is actually a successful marriage of anaerobic and aerobic pathways of metabolism.

Now for that old curse again: "The ratio of fast-twitch to slow-twitch fibers is genetically determined, and cannot be changed by training," say Hatfield and Krotee. You can be sure Carl Lewis's muscle biopsies would be predominantly fast-twitch type, so splendidly suited as he is for the anaerobic 100-yard dash or split-second long jumps. Put another way, certain sports favor the genetic gift of certain types of muscle fibers.

A basic rule is the law of use and disuse—the "use it or lose it" premise. It means that through increasing amounts of stress (work), your muscles gain in strength and endurance. This is basically what weight training is all about. The goal of strength training is to provide a delightful balance by promoting an ideal union of resistance, repetition, and specificity.

Be Specific for Effective Strength Training

Unlike aerobic training, where any work that gets your heart rate up is okay, strength training is highly specific—that is, certain exercises strengthen certain muscle fibers, but not necessarily others. It pays, therefore, to decide in advance the purpose of your strength training: long-distance running, power lifting, or just toting your kids around the park.

Most men are not in search of the sculptured torso of the bodybuilder who approaches his total-body workout with the "curls for the girls" and perfect big muscles idea. Instead, most men are probably simply in search of ways to enhance muscular endurance to carry on life's requirements with a fitter and stronger body.

What kind of strength training should you do?

It depends. Are you going to participate in a sport? If so, your strength goals should probably be sport specific. Such strength training can increase your performance and protect you from injury. Surprisingly, strengthening rarely used parts of your body together with their complementary muscles can better protect you from injury.

If you're athletic, in-season strength training should be maintenance oriented—that is, you should cut down from three or four times a week of your building cycle back to two. On the other hand, it's OK during the off-season to try alternate ways to maintain a strength-training regimen. If summer is your active time, try shoveling snow or working out at the YMCA during winter months. If you're a winter exerciser, summer can offer such simple joys as mowing the lawn.

If you're a member of a gym or health club, perhaps a consultation with an exercise specialist or kinesiologist (an expert on movement) can help you design a sport-specific routine. Coaches and teammates in your sport should have lots of information to help you along as well.

The bottom line is to remain active, but don't forget to rest as well. In addition to health club types of exercise, you can work at such eclectic alternative forms of exercise as gathering maple syrup in the spring thaw, chopping wood during the winter, or hauling dirt and rocks in a wheelbarrow at your summer cabin. Although admittedly not necessarily specific to your particular sport, these activities are all to the good mentally and physically and also offer fruit for your labor.

For power development, you again need to consider the specific motions of your sport. For example, cross-country skiers can develop power by wearing weight vests while performing jumping movements such as hill-bounding. This helps to build the explosive power for the strides they will use during the ski season. Weight vests are also great on long hikes to help build endurance.

Don't be rigid. Throw in a tennis game to improve your agility. Try ballroom dancing or aerobics at the Y. Too much specific training can be boring. Everybody needs a little fun to keep up his or her motivation. Change that old cliché from "No pain, no gain" to "Have fun!"

Making Sure You Do It

But how are you going to design a strength, power, and endurance program if you are an average Joe chained to a job eight hours a day?

You have choices. Rig up a weight training center somewhere in or around your house. If you travel on business, throw one of those rubber band exercisers into your suitcase. Play with the kids: Kids have to be lifted and held. Do something, do anything.

If you've developed some of the eighties mentality, sure, join a health club. That's one way to motivate yourself to get out and exercise. Maybe every time you pay the monthly fee you'll remember to go to the club. Besides, some people prefer the sociability of the gym, replete with hard rock, lycra, communal sweat, and aerobicizing male and female beauties captured by floor-to-ceiling mirrors.

Join a class that meets at certain times. Knowing that you have a karate class every Tuesday and Thursday at lunchtime (and that you've already paid for it) will be a powerful inducement to show up.

How you choose to exercise is a personal matter. Often, it helps to vary where you work out, so this thrice-weekly ritual never becomes boring or stale. Remember, it's the long haul that counts.

Aerobic Workouts

In recent years, the watchword of fitness has been aerobics—running, biking, cross-country skiing, and swimming. Cardiovascular health from aerobic exercises as well as strength training may help to determine not only the length of your life but also the quality and degree of physical activity you may be able to maintain. Aerobic health is unquestionably linked to virtually everything else going on with our bodies.

Maintaining aerobic fitness is principally a matter of regularly working your aerobic drivers—that is, having your heart and lungs work hard routinely. Working your body aerobically, you will maintain a high degree of cardiovascular capacity as well, translated out as endurance capacity.

Here are some recommendations for accomplishing this.

How Hard Should I Exercise?

Generally, the sports medicine gurus advocate three aerobic sessions a week of 30 minutes or more at 65 to 75 percent of your maximal heart rate. Physiologically, this translates to working out well below your anaerobic threshold (the point at which your muscles start to burn from lactic acid overload) and certainly below your maximal heart rate (defined as 220 minus your age). In short, exercise in the comfort zone.

An opposing concept outlined by Ken McAlpine is simply that athletes would be better off using less time but more effort. He advocates high-intensity workouts. Supporting this theory is the opinion held by some exercise experts that a successful method of reversing or preventing aging is by doing high-intensity exercise. McAlpine contends that by following his formula, we can exercise less (albeit harder) at a higher target heart rate.

Bjorn Lasserud, a Minneapolis house painter and perennial world champion in cross-country skiing in his age group—he is now over 70— just doesn't have the time for 3-hour workouts. So Bjorn trains at only three intensities: hard, harder, and quick, get the wagon! Taking into consideration that he was fortunate enough to have picked the right parents, it's still impressive that he has won so many world championship titles in the toughest aerobic sport of them all just by following the "harder is better" concept.

Which path is correct? Perhaps both. Where actual athletic competition is concerned, it's hard, if not impossible, to have that extra competitive edge without some guts-out, high-intensity work. Is it possible to be fit without high-intensity workouts? Yes. Is it possible to compete in your age group and at high levels without it? Probably not. Here again you must explore your goals. If you just want fitness, health, and longevity, then go for the regularity and not all that high intensity.

Actually, knowing how hard you're exercising can be relatively easy. You can buy an expensive Finnish heart rate monitor to wear on your wrist that records your heart rate from the sensor strapped around your chest. By wearing this device, athletes find that they can monitor exercise intensity by listening to the comforting beep of their hearts on this device. If your heart rate drops below the lowest effective exercise intensity or leaps over your anaerobic threshold (when exercise actually becomes detrimental rather than helpful), you know it right away by the signal. The more sophisticated devices can be plugged in to a computer and your workout logged graphically, and even later critiqued as Olympic-level athletes routinely do.

This kind of monitor can be a lifesaver to keep you from "going under" while exercising or, for the competitive types, save you from self-destructing during your first race of the season. The principle of monitoring your heart is actually modeled after phase three cardiac rehabilitation programs in which patients are monitored to keep them from overdoing exercise and to detect any rhythm disturbances during or immediately after exercise.

Many athletes, the types who keep intricate training logs, will routinely record their morning pulse. If it's low, they know they're not overtraining. A high rate indicates that the athlete could be overtired, overtrained, getting sick, or reacting to a medication that could jack up his or her resting heart rate.

A heart rate monitor can be a useful tool. Or it can be overkill. For example, wearing the monitor to bed while having sex could be carrying things a bit too far.

Aside from expensive machines, there are other ways to know if you're exercising at the right intensity. Check your morning pulse before getting up. If it's over 100, for example, you could be getting ill or overtraining. Stopping your exercise to check your pulse rate is one of the simplest methods. Or use the conversation method outlined earlier; that is, you should be able to talk while you're exercising. This is another reason exercise buddies can be such a great idea. If you can continue to carry on your repartee, then you're most likely not over your anaerobic threshold. If you're too winded to speak, you are and should slow down.

A reminder: Someone relatively new to exercise should not begin at high intensity without a complete physical examination that includes a maximal stress test. This is also a convenient way to determine your target heart rate.

Where to Exercise

Some men like to have attractive, nubile, fair-tressed maidens glowing alongside them on the next exercycle. Others feel more comfortable working out with guys grunting in cutoffs, possibly sporting a two-days' beard, and replete with hairy armpits peeping out of Everlast sweatshirts. You may prefer a structured program like the ones the American Lung Association has designed for someone who wants to complete a ski or road marathon but doesn't know how to get started.

Sometimes there's strength in numbers. That's why many people find it helpful having training buddies who can make their running, in-line skating, skiing, or biking go faster (and feel less painful) with mind-consuming banter. Someone out there besides your mother or wife is there to shame, cajole, or intimidate you into maintaining your program and can actually make your new agenda work. Exercise buddies can actually be a healthy form of group therapy. An easy conversation while jogging can keep you from going anaerobic and may help you complete your appointed task.

When to Exercise

One resourceful friend who worked in a ski shop all day did the majority of his skiing at five o'clock in the morning wearing a headlamp designed for miners or Scandinavians, who have very little sun to mix with their snow. Everyone has their own diurnal rhythm, and there are parts of the day when each person is at his or her best. Think about it. You probably have a very good idea about when your body and mind are at their best. Listen to it because that could be the best time to exercise.

A little-known fact is that the largest surge of cortisol and testosterone occurs at four o'clock in the morning and while you sleep. There are probably lots of perfectly good, obsolete reasons why this should be so. It is, of course, the best time to hunt. A good run and chase before breakfast is how we used to dissipate the hormones. So why not exercise early? No sense arriving at your morning staff meetings with your testosterone on high when you can arrive in endorphin heaven with seratonin aplenty.

Most people can find one excuse or another for their failure to find time to exercise: "My lunch break is too short.... I can't change back into my natty work clothes.... I'm too sweaty.... It takes me an hour to cool down.... There is no shower at work...." These may become self-serving excuses. If this is the way you want to live, then the time will come when you can no longer get out of your chair. You won't have the choice of exercising because you physically won't be able to.

Trainers

It is said that you are your own best coach. Although trainers and coaches are sometimes indispensable, you ultimately know your own body best.

One of the greatest athletes of all time, cross-country skiing marathoner Thomas Wassberg of Sweden, reputedly did not keep a training log later in his racing career. He had been training and racing for so long that he didn't need one. Why? He knew his body and knew how to listen to what it told him. You too can get to be like Wassberg just by learning over the years how your body works.

The rest of you may need a pulse monitor to begin to understand which activities make you redline (go over your anaerobic threshold), which ones put you correctly into 65 to 85 percent of your maximum rate range, and which ones aren't quite strenuous enough.

Some athletes like having a coach or trainer; others hate them. If you have a potential problem with criticism, choose your trainer carefully or don't choose one at all. After all, your workouts are supposed to be escapes from stress, not contributors. If you find a trainer who can guide you without setting off these alarms, hold onto him. If it's a she, consider marriage. On the other hand, all you might need is a knowledgeable training partner who can keep you on the right track.

A trainer remains detached from the pain and stress of your middle-aged life. Theoretically, he or she should remain objective about yours. There is a tendency among athletes for us to do a lot of what we know best or enjoy the most. The advantage to having a trainer is that he or she can tell you when you need to take a few days off because you are becoming "sour," or look you straight in the eye and say, "Get off your bleeping butt and do an interval workout." Keep in mind that there aren't too many of us who like to feel the pain of an interval workout, myself included.

Rest

So how do you plan your workouts? There seems to be plenty of evidence that your middle-aged body needs more rest than your teenage son's. That's why many who design master's level training programs will give you two or three days off a week. The ACSM advocates three to four aerobic days plus two to three strength days a week. But you may still choose to combine aerobic with strength exercises on any one day so that you still can find adequate rest time.

Some top-level greats say that they must exercise special care lest they make their workouts into a kind of stew—a hodgepodge of intervals, long slow distance, weight lifting, and so on. It's important to develop a coherent program, stick with it, and not let the whims of the moment turn your program into a planless goulash. Whatever you do, go slowly and increase your exercise in small increments, possibly under the watchful eye of a knowledgeable trainer.

In any case, remember that you're suspended between two contradictory needs. The first is the need for occasional rest. The other is the need to be able to do your workout even when you don't feel like doing it. Your success at conditioning will be the consequence of how well you can walk that fine line.

Just remember, your best strategy is to design a good plan and stick with it. With experience, you'll begin to know instinctively when you should rest and when you shouldn't. Your body can play tricks on a mind that may have lost control. Push too fast, too far, too often, and you could run the risk of overuse injuries or burnout. Typically, overtrained people think that just a little more intensity will kick them out of the doldrums, when what's actually happening—a rapid pulse, unexplained fatigue, or even depression—suggests they are instead in need of rest.

Listen to your body. It often knows what your head will never understand.

When to Get a Stress Test

There is plenty of controversy in this area. If you're running at less than 60 percent of your target heart rate and are below 40 years old, a stress test is superfluous unless you have such cardiac risk factors as smoking, high cholesterol, diabetes, a strong family history of heart disease, or high blood pressure. Obesity, like a sedentary lifestyle, is not a risk factor per se, though it is often accompanied by other high-risk factors.

For the over-40 crowd, some experts advocate skipping a stress test if you have no risk factors. I believe, however, that anyone who plans to push to his maximal heart rate should get tested. Alternatively, either an echo stress or a radioactive study such as a Cardiolyte stress test is in order. If your stress test is positive, fortunately, we now have access to several noninvasive tests (those not requiring entering arteries with needles or catheters) such as a stress echo, a thallium (Cardiolyte) test, or a Dipyridamole stress exam to determine if your stress test is a false positive.

Elite athletes may consider obtaining a VO_{max} exam, which can determine a mysterious number called the anaerobic threshold, the break point, or the lactate threshold—a fancy way of pinpointing when your muscles turn to mush. Put simply, this is the point where lactic acid takes over, making your muscles really cramp and hurt. Lactic acid is the breakdown product of muscle oxidation that accumulates in your body when your muscles can no longer get enough oxygen. The resulting burning sensation is the statement that your muscles have moved into the realm of inefficient metabolism.

Determining your anaerobic threshold has more value than determining your absolute peak or VO_{max}. The ultimate goal is to kick up that elusive anaerobic threshold (break point) to as close as is physiologically possible to your VO_{max}, essentially making your body maximally efficient. Should you become frustrated because you just can't seem to reach the maximal output to which you aspire, remember that the ultimate secret of success in high-level athletic endeavors may still rest in whether you have chosen the right parents.

Signs and Symptoms of Overdoing It

If after exercise you notice the following symptoms, something's wrong:

Immediate
- angina (chest discomfort)
- light-headedness or confusion
- nausea or vomiting
- burning leg pain
- pallor or an ashen color
- labored breathing persisting for more than 10 minutes
- inappropriately slow (or fast) heart rate
- decrease in systolic blood pressure

Delayed
- prolonged fatigue for 24 hours or more
- insomnia
- weight gain due to fluid retention from salt and water overload
- persistent rapid heart beat (tachycardia)

There are times when less is better. If you show any of these symptoms, take heed. You may have overdone it. Stop whatever you are doing and rest! Think seriously about a visit to your favorite sports-minded physician. It may be just as important to listen to your body in the short run than to wait for delayed signs and symptoms of excessive effort.

If you're feeling really rotten or having trouble exercising, don't hesitate to consult a physician. Find a health care provider who understands the dedication you have as an athlete, or your fears as a neophyte fitness buff. There are an increasing number of sports medicine practitioners who specialize in (or are at least knowledgeable about) issues having to do with exercise. They are often your best, but by no means your only, resource.

Another important consideration is to have readily available medical help should you have a problem. Convenience and access to such a facility may determine where you decide to exercise. It doesn't hurt to tell friends where and when you go out for a run. Recent advances in technology make it easy to attach your personal medical identification directly to your running shoes, bicycle, or ski poles. Wear an alert medallion if you have diabetes or a heart condition. Avoid exercising when it is too hot, too humid, or too cold and use good judgment regarding how hard you push yourself. Remember that plenty of fluids such as plain water are essential before, during, and after prolonged exercise. Don't neglect to replenish your carbohydrate stores, especially after a hard workout. Try to select a healthy complex carbohydrate whenever possible.

Weather and Climate Concerns

Working out in any unfamiliar or challenging environment takes acclimatization. For example, adapting to heat may require that you spend some time expanding your plasma volume and learn to increase your rate of sweating so that you can improve your circulatory control. Thus you can ultimately preserve a stable core temperature and heart rate response to any temperature-humidity level regardless of how hard you exercise. Remember to watch your heart rate more closely in very hot and humid circumstances.

Many problems can arise as you pass into the high and very high risk categories of heat exhaustion. They include the following:
- benign but painful heat cramps
- lethargy, anxiety, or irritability due to dehydration (even a 5 percent weight loss can trigger dehydration)
- heat exhaustion due to an internal heat load when the body temperature is over 103°F
- heat stroke (which is sometimes tough to distinguish from heat exhaustion) when the body temperature rises over 106°F, producing nervous system problems

Exercising in the cold actually causes fewer injuries than the same exertion in extremely warm or humid conditions. That's not to say that acclimatizing to the cold doesn't count for something. Someone from Arkansas, whose idea of hell may be 4 inches of fresh powder at 20 degrees, is more likely to develop frostbite than someone who grew up making snow igloos in his backyard in Buffalo, New York. That Buffalo kid's body simply learned how to adjust to the cold. However, many of us who played in the snow throughout our youth also have the tendency to feel our hands and feet get colder and more uncomfortable faster.

Keep exposed skin well covered with creams and the rest of you with breathable, wind-resistant clothing—including a wind shield sewn into your underwear. Frostbite sets in soon after frostnip and represents crystallization of water within your exposed tissues. The freeze may be tolerable, but the rewarming can be excruciating. I know: I've frozen the business end of my penis one too many times in ski races. Never again!

Sweating may help to regulate your body temperature when you're exercising, but once you stop, that same moisture may cause you to continue to lose too much heat. This is when you may develop hypothermia. The latest exercise gear now available lets your body adjust with one-way breathable fabrics, two-way zippers, and flaps and vents for wicking and venting sweat from your skin to your outermost garment so that you won't end up getting hypothermic. New waterproof yet breathable garments make sense because they don't require that you remove any layers to stay dry and warm. Though these duds are highly wind resistant, they permit your sweat to dissipate to the outer air even while you're battened down to keep warm when you stop.

EVERYONE NEEDS TO EXERCISE

There is a certain ethic found in rural America that unfortunately still prevails but deserves challenging. It goes, "If you have to exercise at the end of the day, then you haven't worked hard enough." Maybe this used to be true when farming wasn't mechanized. Now, you're nobody unless your tractor cab has air-conditioning, a sound system, even a cellular phone. Farmers need sensible, coherent exercise just as much as anybody else—possibly more. Theirs is as mentally demanding a profession as any, and they are not immune to stress or tension. That's why you may even see more farmers than ever making time to walk briskly along remote farm roads after a long day in a tractor cab. The alternatives run from standard heart disease to what in Minnesota we call the Stearns County Syndrome—that fortunately rare occasion when an overstressed farmer wakes up on some depressing November morning and shoots his entire family.

Designing an Exercise Program

The American College of Sports Medicine has devoted a lot of space in its *Resource Manual for Guidelines for Exercise Testing and Prescription* to "exercise programming." Studies of compliance in clinical exercise programs reveal dropout rates of around 12 percent at 3 months and as high as 87 percent by 12 months.

I've already talked about such pre-exercise assessment as stress tests and the importance of warm-up and cooldown periods, not to mention stretching and flexibility exercises. These should reflect the intensity of the conditioning program you will engage in. Why? It's simple. Warm-ups and stretching allow your body to adapt to the physical exertion that it will soon encounter.

Group Activities or Lone Wolf?

Here are the primary categories of exercise types that you can adopt. You can go for one style or a combination of styles. There is no right way—what works for you, especially if it keeps you exercising, is OK.

Exercise authority Michael G. Giese, MS, highlights (1) individual exercise, (2) group activities, and (3) circuit techniques. The individual-exercise approach may benefit from a prescription from either an exercise specialist or your coach for improved swimming, blading, hiking, or bowling. Your doctor's advice can be based, to some extent, on your performance during your stress test, what he or she knows about your past number of hours or intensity of your training history, or, if you're the competitive type, on your prior performance at different levels of competition.

However, group activities may keep you honest and get you out there moving. There is nothing like a training partner to lure you away from the desserts and into your jock, running shorts, and shoes. Giese points out that when it comes to group exercising, you should have a higher ratio of leaders to participants if the majority of you out there sweating are beginners. The American Lung Association Runner's Club (or its ski and hiking equivalents) makes maximal use of willing seasoned volunteers who will emphasize learning the right techniques and takes this concept furthest by successfully preparing runners for running or skiers for marathons.

These programs have been successful in developing maximum efficiency while gradually building endurance. There is hardly a way to describe the sense of accomplishment for a middle-aged professional, or a 50-year-old homemaker whose kids have all finished college as he or she completes a first skiing or running marathon. It can be making the impossible possible. In the process, participants shed bad habits such as smoking, inappropriate and excessive drinking, or poor sleeping or eating patterns.

Circuit techniques run the gamut of gut-wrenching outdoor courses combining an aerobic run before, between, and after specific strength exercises such as pull-ups, jumping jacks, stair steps, push-ups, and incline sit-ups. Alternatively, you can run through a series on several Nautilus machines each with a specific strength-training effect. For instance, skiers who want aerobic benefits plus strength will emphasize working the upper body with low weights and high repetitions (my personal favorite).

In developing an exercise program, it is important to create your own personal goals; otherwise, you'll find you lack reasons to don those flimsy shorts, tennies, and T-shirt. Remember those figures about attrition. Keep repeating, "Habit, habit, habit, habit," because your new adventure may not be easy. Try to keep it fun and varied.

Exercise Machines

Sure, there are implicit dangers to bicycling outdoors. Likewise, the indoor equivalent, a stationary bike, has the risk of quickly becoming boring or, for others, allowing you to overexert yourself. A Type A person (like me) will try to compete even on a stationary bike.

The NordicTrack has become a convenient indoor fitness device for millions. A study among University of Minnesota cross-country ski racers (Brad Bart, myself, and Arthur Leon) found that the NordicTrack offered a statistically significant lower perception of exertion than the treadmill. Each demonstrated comparable VO_{max}, but the 11 racers tested could achieve a higher anaerobic threshold—the point where their lactate levels began to climb—on the NordicTrack.

In other words, not only did their muscles get less tired, but they also did not feel they were working as hard. Perhaps they enjoyed it more or became less bored. (Let's not forget they were skiers.) Another benefit of an exercise machine (compared, let's say, with free weights) for strength training is that it can help reduce the chance that you will exercise in the wrong way. That's the very essence of isokinetic exercise—the ability to isolate individual muscles and put them through a preset, highly accurate and effective work load. The beauty of the Nautilus machine, for example, is that it limits the motion to a specific muscle being worked, resulting in a controlled and easily quantified amount of exercise. That is, of course, if you breathe right and avoid muscle-wrenching ballistic movements.

But you don't necessarily have to get all that fancy. Squaw Valley mountaineer-adventurer-filmmaker Eric Perlman carries one of those rubber band–type exercisers (actually a thick version of surgical tubing) on the road with him whenever he travels. He swears by it and still leads 5.12 climbs (very difficult) on California granite.

So what am I going to recommend to our possibly reluctant 40-year-old male neophyte exerciser? A graduated walking program can be the easiest way to start, especially if accompanying someone else offers some much-needed socializing. Should there be a lower-extremity problem, then non-weight-bearing activities such as cycling (stationary, road, or all-terrain), swimming, and chair or floor exercises may be a viable 30 to 40 minute alternative to a hot run in the midday sun. After all, "only fools and Englishmen go out in the midday sun" (and me—I like to exercise at midday).

"THEY'RE HAVING A BALL"

Remember the medicine ball of 100 years ago? Barry Franklin, PhD, director of cardiac rehabilitation and exercise at William Beaumont Hospital's unique Cardiac Rehabilitation Program, has developed ball playing to an art form using unique and playful upper-body activities with different-sized balls described in his innovative manual, On the Ball: Adult Fitness and Cardiac Rehabilitation Programs (Carmel, IN: Benchmark Press, 1990; $19.95, 189 pages). The value of Franklin's book is nicely summed up in one of his introductory quotes: "Next time you pass a children's playground, stop and listen. Hear the laughter? They're having a ball."

The message? You can have fun, too.

Rules for Success

1. Frequency. Increasing exercise to a five-day-a-week program can reinforce the habit part of your formula. Exercise is easier to stay with if you regularly and habitually do it almost every day rather than only a few times a week. There are also physical reasons: The endurance and flexibility you develop can be maintained more easily by frequent exercise. Keep in mind that (active) rest becomes more important as well with age. Likewise, alternating hard with easy exercise, short with long, can build, rather than break down, muscles. And remember: You don't have to punish yourself. Even a good walk after dinner constitutes exercise. Do what you can so that exercise is your escape and relaxation, and not another job or stress producer.

2. Duration. Aim for 20 to 40 minutes of endurance activity each time you exercise. You can increase or decrease the duration depending on the intensity of the activity you choose on any particular day. The high-intensity approach may work if you can only squeeze out a half hour for your exercise.

3. Intensity. If you have any risk factors for heart disease, whoever designs your program should calculate an appropriate heart rate based on the Karvonen formula (see below) as well as an appropriate MET level. (The metabolic equivalent unit [MET] is used to estimate the metabolic cost of your physical activity. One MET = 3.5 milliliters of oxygen consumed per kilogram of body weight per minute.) An exercise prescription can be calculated using your maximal and resting heart rates if, for instance, you are on certain medications. Medications are generally not known to limit your ability to train. Those that affect your baseline heart rate are figured into the Karvonen formula.

THE KARVONEN FORMULA

Normally, target maximal heart rate is figured by the following formula:

220 minus your age = maximal heart rate in beats per minute (BPM)

The Karvonen formula is used to calculate a safe target heart rate during exercise if you are on a medication that alters your natural heart rate. Here is the formula:

$$\begin{array}{r} \text{Normal maximal heart rate (NMHR)} \\ - \text{Normal resting heart rate (NRHR)} \\ \hline \text{Heart rate reserve (HRR)} \\ \times \text{\% of target heart rate (stipulated by your doctor)} \\ \hline \text{Target of heart rate reserve} \\ + \text{Resting heart rate} \\ \hline \end{array}$$

Target maximal heart rate

Let's say you're 56 and happen to be on a beta-blocker such as propranalol (Inderal), a drug that lowers both resting and maximal heart rate, used for hypertension, migraines, or angina. Normally, your target maximal heart rate would be

$$220 - 56 = 164 \text{ BPM}$$

This is how you would figure your target maximal heart rate:

$$\begin{array}{r} \text{Maximal HR} = 135 \text{ BPM} \\ - \text{Resting HR} = 55 \text{ BPM} \\ \hline \text{HR reserve} = 80 \text{ BPM} \end{array}$$

Your doctor says you should be exercising at a 70 to 85 percent maximal exertion range. Thus:

$$\begin{array}{r} 70\% \times 80 \text{ BPM (HR reserve)} = 56 \text{ BPM} \\ + \text{Resting HR 55 BPM} \\ \hline \text{Target maximal HR} = 111 \text{ BPM} \end{array}$$

$$\begin{array}{r} \text{And: } 85\% \times 80 \text{ BPM (HR reserve)} = 68 \text{ BPM} \\ + \text{Resting HR 55 BPM} \\ \hline = \text{Target maximal HR} = 123 \text{ BPM} \end{array}$$

Therefore, your target maximal heart rate should be between 111 and 123 BPM instead of the normal 164 BPM.

Although most medications don't improve exercise capacity, certain ones, such as steroids, can develop greater muscle bulk and hasten muscle recovery after exercise. Yet in no circumstances do I recommend steroids as a muscle or strength enhancer. Their long-term "positive" effects, which have been well documented in the popular press, are far too dangerous.

4. Progression. Fitness does not come overnight. You must gradually increase your activity level. A conservative amount of time to attain a livable level of fitness (from moderate to vigorous exercise) may be about 4 weeks. In older individuals, that may increase to 2 months. An interesting note to this, however, according to John Bland, MD, emeritus professor of medicine and rheumatology at the University of Vermont, himself a marathon runner and masters skier, is that relative youngsters in their forties or younger get out of condition faster (in a matter of a fortnight) compared with the impressive staying power (as long as a month) of people in their sixties to eighties.

He Who Exercises Last, Exercises Best

Overall, a good fitness program benefits everyone. It was true when we were kids; it is true as we reach midlife and beyond. An older individual has as much to gain from strength and aerobic training as anybody in his teens, twenties, or thirties. In the next chapter, you'll find specific techniques to help you continue being a jock well into your twilight years. You are invited.

SUGGESTED READINGS

Blair, Steven N. *Resource Manual for Guidelines for Exercise Testing and Prescription.* Lea and Febiger, 1988. 436 pp.

Chichester, Brian. *Men's Health.* Rodale Press, 1996. 170 pp.

Darville, Fred T., Jr. *Mountaineering Medicine: A Wilderness Medical Guide.* Wilderness Press, 1992. 101 pp.

Franklin, Barry A. *On the Ball: Innovative Activities for Adult Fitness and Cardiac Rehabilitation Programs.* Benchmark Press, 1990. 189 pp.

Hatfield, Frederick and March Hatfield. *Personalized Weight Training for Fitness and Athletics.* Kendall/Hunt, 1984. 191 pp.

McArdle, William D. *Exercise Physiology.* Lea and Febiger, 1986. 696 pp.

Morton, John. *Don't Look Back.* Stackpole Press, 1992. 258 pp.

Peterson, James A. *The Sexy Stomach.* Leisure Press, 1983. 80 pp.

Sacks, Michael H. *Psychology of Running.* Human Kinetics, 1981. 279 pp.

Sheehan, George A., MD. *Running and Being.* Simon and Schuster, 1978. 256 pp.

Wilkerson, MD, ed. *Hypothermia, Frostbite, and Other Cold Injuries.* The Mountaineers, 1986. 105 pp.

Geoff Tabin, M.D.

Physician-Adventurer

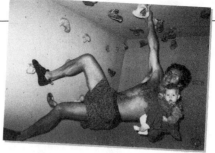

"Above the forty-foot rock obstacle known as the Hillary Step, unadulterated joy welled up inside of me. I knew that I was (finally) going to reach the summit.... Chomolungma (Mount Everest) teased me with several more false summits before the ridge dropped sharply away. The world spread out beneath me. I spent fifteen minutes savoring life as the highest person on earth, alone on the six-foot-by-three platform of ice that is the top of the world."

So writes Dr. Geoff Tabin in his 1993 book, *Blind Corners: Adventures on Seven Continents.* If there ever were a real-life Indiana Jones, Geoff might be the guy. As an undergraduate at Yale, he was already scaling some of the world's highest peaks, including the north face of Carstensz Pyramid (16,023 feet) in Irian Jaya, Indonesia.

Graduating from Yale and the Harvard Medical School—and, by the way, also studying at Oxford—Geoff went on to build a career in ophthalmology, specializing in corneal surgery. But he didn't start his practice right away: Climbing came first. "Back then, I didn't have a penny to my name. I stayed debt free at $12,000 a year."

After five years of gallivanting from peak to peak, Geoff realized it was time to get on with his career. Yet as he was becoming a successful eye surgeon, he always left plenty of time for climbing. Indeed, he has admirably mixed his life's work with his life's passion, teaching cataract surgery at the University of Vermont and in such diverse locations as the Himalayan Eye Institute and, most recently, Pakistan—while still taking on the world's highest peaks. As well as multiple attempts at Everest, he's climbed Mount Kenya in Africa, Vinson Massif in Antarctica, Mount Kilimanjaro in Africa, Mount McKinley in Alaska, Cerro Aconcagua in South America, and Mount Elbrus in Georgia (in the former Soviet Union).

Drawing on the philosophies of both East and West, Geoff cites as his inspirations Goethe, his Sherpa guides ("They do not preach a way of life, they just live it"), and "Boy George" Lowe, America's greatest mountaineer, who was breaking through winter mountain barriers in his mid-fifties. Still, Geoff admits that as he surges into his forties, he has to slow down a bit. Thus, he finds himself turning back to another old love, tennis. At Yale he had been on the tennis team, and the best player at that. Today he's parlayed that skill into playing at the Vermont Men's State

Open Division. "I keep having fun," he says, "but I'm still climbing. I plan to keep on climbing for my whole life."

As he approaches his fifties, this 5'10" 165-pounder divides his life between his practice at the University of Vermont and climbing. And he's still heavily involved in the Himalayan Cataract Project, where he trains the local doctors on how to repair cataracts. "The local physicians there have only two to three years of general medical training after high school," he says, "and I speak a little of the language."

Meanwhile, Geoff has taken up a significant new adventure, raising a family. In his forties, he married a woman with three children and became a father in his own right. One would think that this would put some wrinkles in the travel plans of this seven-continent adventurer. Not so, for Geoff's travel agenda still makes a Bedouin seem as if he's under house arrest.

Although other men may live lives of quiet desperation, Geoff keeps looking for new adventures. As he so eloquently sums up a simple philosophy for a complex life: "The most difficult obstacles to surmount in climbing, as in life, are mental."

Amen.

Chapter 8

Practical Techniques
■ **Stretching, Strength, and Aerobics**

> In a man's middle years there is scarcely a part of the body he would
> hesitate to turn over to the proper authorities.
>
> E. B. White, "A Weekend With the Angels"

If you've read this far, you've no doubt decided to start or reinvigorate your
exercise regimen on the assumption you will improve your health and
brighten your long-term physical outlook. At this point, I will assume
that you have no physical inhibitors to taking up a more strenuous
lifestyle and that you are psychologically ready to go.

For any of a number of reasons, it is important to take this step by step
to achieve the best results, to remain free from injury, and to avoid trig-
gering a backlash by your body. Thus, I will start at the beginning with
preparatory steps and take you through the process.

PREPARING TO EXERCISE

Plan to drink plenty of water. H_2O bathes all your tissues, maintains
cardiovascular volume, and ensures proper blood flow to all your muscles.
Such liquid consumption does not translate out to beer, wine, or coffee.
Water means water!

Avoid eating just before exercise. Eating tends to pull important
blood from your muscles and heart into your gut, leaving the rest of your
body hungry for nourishment and oxygen.

Stretching

Before starting organized exercising, you need to spend time on some
extra special preparation that becomes particularly important as you get
older. (Do as I say, not as I always do. This is one of my weakest areas, and
I pay the price with pulled hamstrings, quadriceps, and you-name-it.) You
must know by now that you may not be as limber as you once were, and

your muscles are more susceptible to becoming overextended or, worse yet, torn. In other words, you need to stretch.

Stretching is not a complicated concept, nor are its benefits that hard to understand. It improves flexibility. Stretching prevents muscle tears and strains and, done the right way, increases the training benefits of your exercise. It also decreases recovery time and injury. Unfortunately, too many people spend too much time exercising and too little time stretching. Bob Anderson, author of *Stretching,* has made a lot of money just by telling a very simple story to athletes of every discipline. What's his new holy writ? Nothing more than clearly describing easy ways to stretch. Much of his secret rests with applying the age-old practice of yoga, which has been around for thousands of years to exercise.

Stretching reaches down to your tiniest muscle fibrils at an ultramolecular level, ultimately enabling big muscle groups to develop more power. This is just another example of how wonderfully the body works—how even the smallest building blocks contribute to the whole organism.

Stretching promotes body awareness. Regular stretching easily shows you where you hurt, where you are becoming stronger, or where you need work. Not only will you reduce muscle soreness, but you should be able to exercise sooner and harder. Adequate stretching during your cooldown also helps massage out painful concentrations of lactic acid from your muscles. You may well even be able to sleep better.

According to Strauch and Ehrich of the Minneapolis Institute of Athletic Medicine, muscles have four properties. They can thicken and shorten, stretch when a force is applied, regain normal size after being stretched, and receive and react to stimuli.

Muscles can stretch to 150 percent of their normal length. This property is crucial to preventing injury because joints, tendons, ligaments, and connective tissues attached to the muscles are not particularly elastic. Enhancing the elasticity of your muscles can protect the more rigid parts of your body from injury. The muscles take up the stress by stretching instead of tearing or breaking.

Stretching is important both before and after your workout, though you can certainly take a shot at stretching almost any time. But no matter when you do it, certain universal rules apply:

1. First, warm up. Ideally, a short five-minute warm-up of a light jog or swim, or five minutes on any form of exercise machine (such as an exercycle), can precede stretching. This allows your muscles to warm up and increases their blood flow. Some folks even duck into a sauna to let the dry heat loosen them up as their heartbeat quickens. The muscles become more pliable, more elastic, and then can be more safely stretched. You can even have your massage.

2. Avoid "ballistic stretching." Remember when it was not uncommon to see your average weekend athlete bobbing up and down touching either toe in a fashion not unlike those oil rigs out in California? Well, those days are past. The purpose of stretching is to avoid any rapid and jerky motions, which may overextend your muscles too quickly, to the point of tearing.

3. Do "static stretches." Here's how: Engage in the stretching maneuver to the point where you feel a significant end resistance (but not pain), and then hold the position for 10 to 20 seconds. No need for you to go beyond this point. You will feel your muscle lengthen as your tiniest muscle fibrils gently pull apart. If you feel any pain in the muscle, you may be stretching too far. Stop stretching that particular muscle group.

4. Don't bounce. Instead, apply a constant pressure until you begin to feel your muscle group stretch. It takes time.

5. Go slow. Back off if you feel any pain. Recall that, with aging, there is a progressive decline in your flexibility.

6. Stretch opposing muscle groups. Systematically stretch and relax different muscles of the body, being sure to stretch opposing muscles—quads versus hamstrings, triceps versus biceps, abs versus back muscles.

7. Don't forget to breathe. Concentrate on breathing through all your stretches, particularly exhaling. Breathe deeply and slowly. Proper breathing will allow you to relax faster and stretch farther.

8. Repeat your stretches. Two to six repetitions of each stretching exercise will do the trick.

9. Stretch regularly. Perform regular stretches at least three times a week even if you're not working out.

The stretches I describe in the following sections are just a few examples of exercises you can perform to increase the elasticity of your muscles.

The Achilles Stretch

The issue here is pure pain. In middle-aged people—and especially men—the large Achilles tendon can become so brittle that a relatively mild strain can literally cause it to snap. I've had friends who have had this happen doing simple things like stepping off a curb. Typically it occurs during or after taking part in a sport in which you are changing direction often and suddenly—tennis and racquetball are favorites that require sudden stops and starts.

The cause, however, doesn't matter. The effect does. The most common reaction is having one or both Achilles tendons snap. In case you're wondering how this feels, it's sort of like being shot in the lower calf. To avoid this happening to you, do the stretches described below several times a week:

- Sit on the ground with your legs straight in front of you. Pull your toes toward you into a frog leg position. Pull for 15 seconds and then relax for 15 seconds. Repeat 5 to 10 times.
- Stand and push against a wall or pole. Move slowly and deliberately as you move one foot farther and farther away from the pole, with the heel flush to the floor. Exert pressure for 15 seconds each time, then relax for the same amount of time. Switch legs so that the other leg is in front as you push. Don't bounce.

Quadriceps and Groin Stretches

The quadriceps ("quads") and groin are two of the most powerful muscles in the human body. As too many men know, a pulled groin muscle really hurts and can take a whole lot of time to heal. Try these exercises to avoid this happening:

- Sit on the ground with your legs apart and gently lower your upper body first over one thigh, then over the other. This will stretch both your quads as well as your hamstrings.
- First pull one ankle, then the other, around to your back and again gently fall backward. Just pull one leg if that is all you can tolerate at first. You can do this standing, one leg at a time. You can feel your muscles stretching. Go slowly and carefully. If it hurts, cut back.
- Lie with your legs apart. You can have a partner push his or her feet against your feet, stretching your groin. Another technique is to have a partner lean full against your back, slowly and gently pushing down to stretch your hamstrings and groin muscles. It is important for partners to immediately signal if they feel any pain.
- Sit with your feet tucked up against your groin. Try (either alone or with assistance) to slowly begin to flatten your knees to the ground on either side.
- One of my favorite stretches, but one that takes quite a bit of balance, is the infamous "pelican stretch." It requires you to stand flat on one leg and bring the fingers to the toes while pulling up on your opposite foot behind your back. The pelican can be performed while holding onto a stable object... such as your wife, girlfriend, or a table. That is, if she's still with you. (The table, I mean.)

Hamstrings

A pulled hamstring can become a most persistent nuisance. Once a hamstring gets injured by being pulled, strained, overextended, or overworked, much time can elapse before it feels normal again. Plus it will have the tendency to pull out more easily in the future.

Of critical importance here is to avoid overstrengthening the opposing quadriceps on the front of your thigh while underworking your hamstring, an imbalance that could predispose you to a hamstring strain.

- While standing, slowly and incrementally move your feet apart as if you are going to do the splits. It helps to wear shoes that grip slightly so that you don't suddenly slip!
- Place first one leg, then the other, on top of a picnic table (for some, anyway, an excellent height) and, without bouncing, gently lower the upper part of your body down over the extended knee, stretching the hamstrings—the muscles at the back of your thigh.
- Sit on the floor and split your legs apart, trying to keep your knees as straight as possible. Gently lower your torso out and over your thighs. Here, too, you can have assistance from someone pushing gently on your back or pulling your arms from the front to maximize your stretch.

Hip Rotators

The hip rotators are often neglected in stretching regimens. Here are two exercises that should keep those hips limber.

- You can also do this with a partner. Sit and let your legs go apart. Have someone you trust hold and push against your feet with their feet. That person can pull your hands as he or she pushes your legs apart. Stop if you feel any discomfort.
- Sit and place your legs far apart to the side, twisting your right leg into a flexed position forward while your back foot is pulled in extension. You can use a table for balance.
- Sit on the floor so that both knees are flush to the ground and extending in the same direction. Separate the knees slightly, with both still flush to the floor. The effect is of half a human pinwheel. Gently twist your body from right to left several times. Repeat with the feet extended in the opposite direction.

Lower Back

The lower back is one of the most easily injured parts of the body, the Waterloo of nearly every middle-aged body. Yet most lower-back pain can be avoided through consistent stretching and exercising into your later years. Too often backs are injured not because they're overused but because they're understrengthened. Some ways of avoiding pain in the lower back include strengthening your abdominal muscles and paying attention to proper posture when standing and (especially) sitting at work or at play.

- Don't slouch.
- Eat your vegetables.
- Avoid sitting in airplane seats.
- If you must sit for a long time in a car, bus, train, plane, or professional conference—or if you spend lots of time in front of the computer, as I do—get out or get up and stretch your back regularly, about once every hour. You won't regret it if you do; you may regret it if you don't.

And do one or more of these stretches three times a week:
- Place your arms as far above your head as you can reach and gently and slowly bring your arms first back then forward. Here again, a partner can assist you in extending your stretch.
- Lie on the floor and sit up enough to gently clasp your ankles. Then slowly unroll your spine from the tailbone up, flattening each point of your spine on the floor as you roll down. Be careful not to overflex your neck. You may also do this exercise with both legs straight, still reaching as far out as you can for your ankles, then rolling. Doing these two stretches will tell you a lot about how flexible you actually are.
- Stand up. Place both your hands on your lower back and now push forward. Lean your upper body back over your hands. This is an easy one to do in the office.
- This is taken from an old yoga stretch called "the lion." Get down on all fours on the ground. With your arms straight, arch your back down, forcing your stomach and chest toward the floor with your head back and up in the air. Lift your head higher and stretch your stomach down like a cat (or lion) in the sun. It feels so good, especially in the morning. Try sticking out your tongue as far as it will go. Roar if you want.
- Lie on your back and lift your legs into the air above you. Gently let them fall down over your head. Do this alone, because your butt will be an irresistible target to mischievous spouses, friends with divided loyalties, or small children.
- Sit on the floor, cross your right foot over your left leg, and flatten it onto the floor. Then reach with your left hand across your body as far to the right as you can comfortably go. Switch legs and repeat this exercise on the other side.

Biceps and Triceps

Even if you have no desire to look like Arnold Schwarznegger, you still need to keep your biceps and triceps limber. You never know when you're going to be called on to lift a child or grandchild, a niece or nephew, a bag of groceries, a garbage can, or a damsel in distress. The following exercises should prepare you for any eventuality:

- Grasp your hand above your head and pull slowly from one side to the other. This will also help to stretch your long back muscles.
- Next, place both hands behind your back and pull first to the left and then to the right, switching grasping hands. This maneuver will stretch your remaining back muscles.

Pectorals

The pecs too can get tight, though looking at your body in the mirror you might not think so. All that sag, my friend, is not firm muscle but flabby muscle or fat. If you think you're a candidate for a brassiere, it's time to tone up those pecs. But first do this stretching exercise:

- If alone, start by holding your arms out from your sides and then slowly, steadily pull them back behind you. Another way is to have a trusted friend gently pull your arms backward. Just remember to tell him or her when to stop.

Trapezius

This is the muscle that is typically traumatized when some pushy son-of-a-yuppie bashes his dad's Beamer into your rear bumper, resulting in your whiplash, not his. Proper stretching ahead of this event can prevent lots of pain and disability:

- Rotate your head in a full 360-degree circuit, stopping every 15 degrees for a contraction of the neck muscles, followed by a relaxation. This stretch is also good for releasing stress.

Facial Muscles

Like your neck muscles, the set of tiny muscles in your face can be key to whether you feel relaxed or jittery. Fortunately, they respond beautifully to 15 seconds of contraction in a forced, overdone smile, a frown, or an all-around scrunch, followed by a relaxation. Try this in front of a mirror and notice the difference between a stressed face and a relaxed face. Get the picture? If you're at all into body language, you'll immediately recognize which "you" looks best.

Years ago, when Western civilization didn't have a clue about the benefits of yoga, photos of facial exercise would be shown as an example of the presumed weirdness of this Eastern discipline. In fact, facial stretching is a far more effective (and certainly less addictive) stress reducer than many of our commonly used drugs—including alcohol.

The better the athlete, the more likely he or she stretches. You're never too fast, too good, or too strong to stretch. This same truth applies equally to back stretches and strengthening exercises. One member of the Norwegian national cross-country ski team, a gold medalist several times over, reputedly spends an hour a day stretching. If you have a massage therapist, he or she can incorporate stretches into your therapy sessions, focusing on what movements your body needs the most. And as I mentioned earlier, many athletes find they can stretch better after warming up in a steam room or sauna. The warmth can successfully loosen up tight muscles and ligaments, allowing them a greater range of movement.

You are never too old to stretch. On the contrary, as you age, stretching the bod becomes even more important.

Designing a Strength-Training System

Finding a strength-training system that suits you can be an art form. What works for an active outdoors person won't necessarily work for somebody who's been a desk jockey for the past several decades.

A couple of reminders before I go further: First, mix and match your exercises by incorporating variety. You'll be better able to work your new program into a busy schedule or family responsibilities you can't always control. Let's face it—membership in a health club isn't the solution if you're on the road two out of every four weeks or just can't find the half-hour necessary to get there, change, work out, shower, and so forth. I'm afraid that I'm a closet changer. I've perfected the fine art of changing in my car without getting arrested for exposure.

Second, don't hesitate to get help. Read books (like this one—a good beginning!) and talk to knowledgeable people. Your local physical therapist or exercise specialist at the gym should be able to design a starting strengthening and aerobics program. The American College of Sports Medicine has a list of exercise specialists who can get you into gear no matter how out of shape you believe you are.

There are almost as many strength-training systems as there are exercisers. Here are some examples:

1. Pyramid: Begin by performing a set of three to five repetitions with a light weight, adding five pounds at a time for each new set. Repeat three to five sets until you poop out.

2. Heavy-to-light: Start with heavier weights and progress gradually to lighter ones. The same goal applies as in pyramiding—that is, exhaustion.

3. Rest-pause: Do maximum weight until failure. (Ouch!)

4. Compound exercise: Combine curling and pressing the weight in one rather than two separate motions.

5. Set: Perform your exercise a given number of times—for example, 10 to 15—rest a few minutes, and then repeat the exercise for the required number of sets you have logged. You can vary this with the super set system, in which you oppose antagonist exercises (each working opposing sets of muscles) back-to-back.

6. Cheater: Arm curls can be real tough if begun with your arms at full extension. However, you can "cheat" by using your thighs to lift your forearms into a position where your biceps can easily take over. It's a good way to help yourself curl heavier weights.

7. "Split" routine: This is more for those gonzo bodybuilding types. They've got so many muscles to develop, bless their narcissistic souls, that they do group 1 (Monday, Wednesday, and Friday) for arms, legs, and trunk and group 2 (Tuesday, Thursday, and Saturday) for chest, shoulders, and back. (Yes, Mother, these tend to be driven types.)

8. Peripheral heart action: The lifter balances one exercise with another far removed from the first to avoid overfatiguing a particular muscle. An example would be following calf lifts with bench presses.

9. Circuit training: This aids in endurance development. A lifter initially uses lighter weights for a set period of time. Then, while maintaining the same weights, the lifter gradually shortens the overall time to complete the exercises.

SAMPLE CIRCUIT TRAINING SCHEDULE

Physical Activity	Duration
Warm-up ■ Exercycle or running in place	5–10 minutes
Stretching	10 minutes
Total exercise duration (12–20 reps, 1–2 sets for all) ■ Bench press or chest press ■ Leg press ■ E-Z curls ■ Leg squats ■ Sit-ups with weight ■ Hip flexors or hanging leg lifts	35–45 minutes
Cooldown Stretching, light calisthenics, cycling, running, relaxation	5–10 minutes

(Thanks to Hatfield and Krotee, *Personalized Weight Training*.)

---

10. Super Circuit: Combines the best peripheral heart action, set, and circuit training systems, allowing a 30- to 45-second aerobic activity (aerobic dance, cycling, NordicTrack, running, or jumping rope) between each station, sequence, or exercise. This is one way to ensure that those of you who are high achievers successfully maintain your target heart rate at 65 to 75 percent of maximum while strength training. The trick here is to combine light weights, relatively high repetitions, and alternate muscle groups.

Taken three times a week for 10 weeks, the super circuit system should increase your lean body mass, increase your biceps girth, and increase your treadmill endurance time, flexibility, strength, and VO_{max}. It also burns approximately 1,100 calories an hour.

Super circuit is not for the faint of heart or frail of body, especially in the back, knee, or shoulder departments. Don't forget the 5- to 10-minute warm-up and cooldown periods before and after as well as stretching. You should actively rest and stretch for two minutes before repeating the (torture) program.

Weight Training Exercises
The Bench Press
Helps: Pecs, deltoids, and triceps

Equipment: Free weights, lifting bench

How to: This exercise is done in a vertical position, either standing or sitting, preferably at a weight bench for safety. The bench press differs from the lying-down bench press, which offers less work to the back muscles and perhaps a bit more to the abdominals.

Take a comfortable position and grip the bar holding the right weights—that is, start light and work up—with your forearms vertical. Be sure your back is in a secure vertical position. Exhale while lifting, inhaling as you return the weights gently back before repeating the movement.

Half Squats
Helps: Glutes (butt muscles), hams (backs of the thighs), quads (those strong front thigh muscles), and the erector spinae group (the little suckers that do most of the work holding up your spine in the lower back). They're also the ones most commonly injured lifting. That's why it's important to learn how to do this properly. Some experts advocate using a lifting belt. One in leather goes for $10 and looks great when you are riding your Harley with that new trophy mama of yours.

Equipment: Free weights, lifting belt, squat machine (optional).

How to: Keep your head up, your feet about shoulder width apart, feet toed out slightly. Exhale as you start with your lower leg at an 80-degree angle to your thighs, back straight as you tighten and straighten your torso out, lifting an appropriate weight (again, start light). Free weights work just fine, but a squat machine is faster and safer because it forces you into the proper lifting position. Inhale on the gentle and slow downward phase (don't go ballistic; no crashes, please, because that's how you can strain your muscles).

Biceps Curls
Helps: Biceps and brachialis group

Equipment: Free weights (either long bar or hand weights) or curl machine (optional)

How to: Go from the palm-up position (flush with the pad, if you're using a machine) while holding the weight. Bring the bar up to your chin on the exhale and return it slowly back to the starting position as you inhale.

Clean and Press
Helps: Erector spinii, glutes, quads, hams, traps, delts, triceps, and the serratus anterior

Equipment: Free weights (long bar), lifting belt, partner to spot (optional, but recommended)

How to: This is the "big kahuna" of all lifts, so important that it's a single Olympic discipline all its own. With the weights on the floor, the lifter grips the bar, palms down, shins 2 inches from the bar. With a graceful movement, the bar is brought up with a straightening and tightening of the back, and a snap of the wrists onto the anterior deltoids of the shoulder. From there it is exhaling all the way home into the mightiest lift of them all, both arms outstretched above your head, forming with your body one powerful victory symbol, the bar capping it all. Again, don't get overly ballistic on the way down or let yourself get caught between the bar, weights, and the floor.

Calf Raises
Helps: Calf muscles, Achilles tendons, feet

Equipment: Free weights, board, step, etc.

How to: This is an easy exercise you can do even without weights on any stairs, curb, or even on a machine (squat machine will do). Back your heels off the board, and raise your body and the weight in a slow deliberate exhale, then return back to a position that prestretches your calf and go for it again, hoisting the weights against a straight back and legs.

Considering the danger we're in at our age of snapping our Achilles tendons, this exercise should be done carefully and only after proper stretching. Yet this doesn't mean neglecting it altogether! I know of a 30-year-old pathologist who popped both his Achilles tendons while running after his kids. Had he stretched regularly, he might have avoided this! But who thinks they have the time. A very type A surgeon friend of mine managed to clip one of his Achilles tendons this way as well.

Dips

Helps: Triceps, anterior delts, pec major and minor, lat dorsi (that long monster down the entire length of your back), and teres major

Equipment: parallel bars or other dip apparatus

How to: Start out suspended from the parallel bars atop straight arms, fingers out, and slowly lower your entire weight until your upper arms are parallel with the floor. Then (here's where it hurts) go back up again. If you like to suffer a bit, try doing this with a weight suspended from your waist. At first, as with chin-ups or pull-ups, a friend can assist you part of the way until you are strong enough to go it alone. You can then also progress to additional weights.

Back Extensions

Helps: Erectors: hamstrings, triceps, gluts, traps, and rhomboids

Equipment: Hand weight (optional), padded exercise board with straps

How to: In the skiing world, this one exercise done fairly religiously either with or without a 10-pound weight behind your neck can make the difference between heaven and hell in your next classic-style 30K ski race. Slip a strong and comfortable area of your calves under the strap and lie prone on the board with your belt right about on the edge of the padded board. Inhale as you drop slowly from a prone position. Go down to the floor at a right angle to your lower body to a 90-degree position to get your money's worth as you extend your elbows out. Then exhale and lift your head up and forward as you return back to the prone position. Remember not to go ballistic on the downstroke. Too rapid drops are frequently where accidents can happen. You know that by now.

Incline Bench Bent-Knee Sit-Ups

Helps: The recti (abdominus: superior and inferior), psoas major (the filet mignon muscle), the pectineus, and the rectus femoris

Equipment: None (incline board optional)

How to: Lie on your back on the floor with your knees raised and your feet flat on the ground. Don't grab the back of your neck to avoid straining it. You can place your arms across your chest if you like. While exhaling, separate your spine, vertebrae by vertebrae, as you would in a floor roll, getting as close as possible when coming up to your knees kept bent at 90 degrees. (Hatfield and Krotee describe it as a motion not very unlike unrolling a carpet.) If you use an incline board, limit the angle of the incline so that you can still do 20 to 25 reps comfortably.

Lat Pulldowns

Helps: Lat dorsi, teres major, rhomboids, and biceps

Equipment: pulldown machine or portable surgical tubing exerciser (popular among the cross-country set)

How to: Kneel in front of, or sit on, the seat of the pulldown machine and slowly draw the bar or tubing handle down either behind your neck or in front of your chin while exhaling. Return slowly. No ballistics! Jerking to your muscles can only cause damage.

Balancing Strength With Aerobic Exercise

One very fit friend notes, "I have exercised all my life and have *never* done weight work." This is coming from someone who did well enough on the competitive Dartmouth ski team to have lettered. He goes on: "Weight work is boring. How could anyone do weight work without some other form of stimulating exercise?"

Good question. And in a way, he's right. Although there are many active ways to gain aerobic conditioning, strength training is another matter. The solution is that you *can* add muscle strengthening to your regular aerobic exercise. For example, you can wear an inexpensive weight vest or ankle weights while walking, biking, climbing mountains, cross-country skiing, playing tennis, or chasing kids or while using a treadmill, rowing machine, or NordicTrack. If biking, periodically pull out that antique Schwinn from the garage and head for a few hills. That'll build the leg muscles. Another option is to replace an often exhausting anaerobic workout (the "faster is better" kind) with what the endurance competitors call "LSD"—long slow distance. Physiologists contend that LSD increases capillarization in your extremities and with it your potential to tolerate or excel in endurance activities.

Even if you're not on a gung-ho regimen to become the world's fittest 50 year old, some form of aerobic exercise at 65 to 85 percent of your VO_{max} could do you a world of good. Put a simpler way, this means you and a friend can exercise while still continuing to chat.

The Ken Cooper Prescription

Dr. Kenneth Cooper, who directs the Cooper Aerobics Center in Dallas and is the author of several best-selling books including the series *Aerobics: The Preventive Medicine* and *The Aerobics Program for Total Well-Being,* made popular the notion of aerobic exercise as a method to happiness, contentment, and maintaining healthy fitness.

Cooper contends from studies he has performed at his center that people who are physically fit are less depressed, have a better self-image, and show a more positive attitude toward life. In *How to Get Back in Shape After 40,* he argues that it's never too tough, too risky, or too late to start an exercise program. Several recent studies continue to support Cooper's original premise that aerobic exercise can improve your health. Cooper advocates a mere 30 minutes of sustained activity, three times a week.

The following is a six-week "starter program" that men over 40 can try, even those with advanced heart disease or after bypass surgery (although we'd recommend running this one by your cardiologist first):

Cycle 1

Weeks 1 to 3: On an empty stomach, walk for 15 minutes, preferably first thing in the morning. Repeat this three times a week or more if possible. Try to walk with your spouse or a friend an hour after dinner.

Week 4: Increase to 20 minutes a session.

Week 5: Increase to 25 minutes each time.

Week 6: Increase your activity to 30 minutes each time. At the same time, you can aim to decrease the time it takes to walk two miles. Cooper advises, "Walk, don't run or jog during this period."

Cycle 2

Only if you are symptom free (no chest pain, shortness of breath, or musculoskeletal pain) can you safely and comfortably move to jogging, aiming to decrease the time it takes you to run two miles first from 30 then to 20 minutes over a 6-week period. "Don't rush into exercise," says Cooper. "It may have taken 20 years for you to get out of shape, and if you try to get back into shape in 20 days, it can be dangerous... or worse yet, potentially fatal."

ALTERNATIVE EXERCISES

If you're extremely overweight or have painful joints that cannot tolerate weight-bearing activities, then exercising in water (aquatics) and swimming may be your métier. Geriatrician Joel Posner, MD, of the Center for Continuing Health at the Medical College of Pennsylvania, Philadelphia, states that although swimming may be fine aerobically, it does not protect against osteoporosis. If you are an avid swimmer, the stairmaster or a low-impact step aerobics program can be excellent alternatives to jogging and lifting as a way to also strengthen your bones and muscles.

Do What You Can

We are all part of a culture that rarely walks, let alone runs. We're not like the Dutch, who bicycle everywhere. The first Hmong immigrants who came to Minnesota became superb soccer players because of how strong their legs were from their habit of walking up and down their native hilly countryside. Norwegians hike, ski, and walk, and they are a healthy people. On the other hand, Americans sit and watch others exercise. Exercise to them means watching huge football players bashing each other around on a field, a modern-day form of gladiatorial combat. Or sitting through a game where most of the time everyone is waiting around for one guy to throw a ball as hard as he can past another guy who's trying to hit it with a thick stick. Are these exercise? Even the so-called active parents who encourage their kids to become involved in team sports sit around in bleachers or folding chairs as their kids run around a field or gymnasium. Notice something wrong here?

It's up to you to change your exercise perspective and become active. Walk the malls with your spouse. Buy a NordicTrack or a treadmill and use them—so that yours does not become just another piece of furniture in the family room, a modern sculpture designed to impress visitors. (Studies seem to show they usually don't.) Kick the soccer ball around with your kid. Do something crazy: Try in-line skating! (In Minneapolis, promoters have opened the Humphrey Metrodome for skaters. The screamers get one building level and the slow set another.) Walk or bicycle to work several times a week. But wear a helmet.

If you're living a rural existence, you can spend several hours a week sawing, chopping, splitting, or storing wood. If you're a city mouse, try mowing your petite lawn with a manual mower. Looking for something to do over your lunch break? Take to the pool for laps. Besides cross-country skiing or rowing, there isn't a better overall exercise for thinning down your body and building aerobic capacity. I personally have never enjoyed chlorinated pools.

If you happen to be an older father and have a new baby, pick up a jogging baby carriage or just a back carrier. Hiking—not riding—around your local golf course with a 15-pound baby strapped to your back can give you plenty of endurance-building exercise. If you're a cross-country ski buff, you can haul along your kid in a Norwegian pulk, a light sled that attaches to the skier with wooden poles. The ingenious sled has a built-in windshield and canvas outer covers to help your child stay warm and doesn't roll over unless you do. Just make sure you remember you're the one who's exercising and not your child. Make sure she or he is properly bundled for the elements.

For the biking set, there are some pretty slick bike trailers replete with wind shields and high-visibility tall flags to make sure you bring your precious cargo home intact to a skeptical wife. (But always remember that each of you must wear a helmet.)

Stairmasters, exercycles, healthriders, treadmills, and other such exercise equipment can be on the pricey side, but look on them as an investment, much like an insurance policy. Their advantage is that they can be readily accessible to you before you leave for work in the morning or at the end of a busy, emotionally exhausting day. One physician I know slides along on his Nordic Track while reading medical journals. Other guys watch the news or read the paper. I'm an outdoors fanatic and don't find reading the newspaper inside a room a suitable escape from the stressors of my life, but if your opportunities are limited, take whichever ones you can get. The bottom line is to get that body moving.

Another option are the circuit courses available in most cities. They allow you to work your own weight against various bars and beams with exercises such as push-ups, pull-ups, balance beam walks, and so forth. A circuit course in a downtown city park can be a welcome respite from an otherwise stressful business trip and can provide an efficient and enjoyable way to fulfill all your exercise needs at the same time. Another advantage of a circuit course is that you can easily measure your time and assess your endurance capacity.

Whatever you choose to do is fine. The important thing, of course, is that you do it.

See you out there.

Kevin Burnside

Pipe Fitter

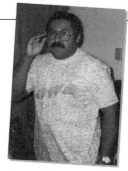

"I pretty much have always exercised," says jour-
neyman pipe fitter Kevin Burnside. Though in his
early forties, he looks more like a 33 year old, a
tribute not only to his fitness but to his decision
to quit drinking some years back.

Kevin spent the early years of his life with his grandmother out in the
country near Pershing, Iowa. His mother had left him there when she
went to the Twin Cities to finish school. While on the farm, he developed
a love for hunting and fishing. Eventually he joined his mother and young
sister in Minneapolis, where he spent the next two decades living near
downtown and the old train station.

Though he liked sports and played basketball in high school in South
Minneapolis, he eventually fell in with the wrong crowd, and drinking
began to occupy a lot of his time. Finally, in his mid-twenties, after a few
blackouts and DWIs, he decided to go into treatment.

Kevin has been off the bottle now for almost 20 years and finds happiness in his work, exercise, family, and friends. Kevin points out that his
work is a major element of staying in shape. "I'm lifting pipes, moving
pipes, walking up and down ladders all day," he says. And though at 5'6"
Kevin would never be mistaken for Wilt the Stilt, basketball has remained
his sport of choice all seasons of the year. He'll hit the courts most any
winter Saturday for a couple hours of pickup ball. Then, when summer
arrives, he's sometimes at the park two to three days a week regardless of
how hard he's been working.

In the diet arena, Kevin admits that getting to work by 7:00 A.M. makes
breakfast tough. The best he can usually do is grab a cup of English tea,
his favorite morning beverage. Without too much guilt, Kevin confesses
that he tends to gravitate toward the cheeseburgers or chicken at lunch.
Supper is when Kevin has plenty of time to sit down with daughters Adra
and April for some of his wife Hazel's fine southern cooking. Fortunately,
despite all the saturated fats and salt that distinguish ethnic African-
American cooking, Kevin reports only a minimal history of hypertension
and hypercholesterolemia. Still, the good southern cooking shows on his
belly, a fact he sheepishly admits.

Like most men, Kevin chooses not to be too concerned about the association between love handles and hypertension or sudden heart attacks.
"Yeah, I'd certainly like to see myself lose some weight and shape up my
stomach," he acknowledges. But other things in life are more important

—like family, work, playing basketball, and his strong belief, he says, "in a higher power."

Much has changed since Kevin's early years on the farm in Iowa, but it's apparent that in his early forties Kevin has a good grip on the process of growing older and his position in this transition.

Chapter 9

Nutrition

■ To Eat or Not to Eat

The History of every major Galactic Civilization tends to pass through three distinct and recognizable phases, Survival, that of Inquiry, and that of Sophistication, otherwise known as the How, Why, and Where phases. For instance, the first phase is characterized by the question, "How can we eat?"; the second by the question, "Why do we eat?"; and the third by the question, "Where shall we have lunch?"

Douglas Adams, *The Hitchhiker's Guide to the Galaxy*

We've all been bombarded by information, hype, and outright fluff regarding nutrition. Everybody's an expert, and everybody has a theory.

We are told these days that everything we've ever been taught about what we eat is wrong. We are told, for example, that the average American diet of 40 percent carbohydrate, 40 percent fat, and 20 percent protein is at the heart, if you'll excuse the pun, of the matter. Robert Haas, who wrote *Eat to Win* and *Eat for Success,* advises we eat 60 percent carbohydrate, 25 percent fat, and 15 percent protein. Dean Ornish, the doctor who wrote *Reversing Heart Disease,* advocates even stricter limitations on fat intake. Dr. William Manahan, former president of the American Holistic Medical Association and author of *Eat for Health,* says diet depends upon body type. For certain individuals, a diet high in complex carbohydrates is great; for others, it causes problems. Some people just need (and can tolerate) higher levels of fat and protein.

So who's right? Hard to say. All we know is that the experts all suggest, to one degree or another, that we totally change the way we eat.

This is all very difficult because what we eat is so much a function of our culture and sense of self. We are constantly bombarded by advertisements for the latest fast-food (some folks say "fat food") hamburger combination. We are told to drink plenty of milk. We are taught that the ultimate dinner out is steak and lobster. We are tempted by slick television commercials to buy prepared foods often high in salt and low in fiber.

On the other hand, there are those who would accuse low- or zero-fat advocates of designing food so dry and tasteless it could be mistaken for dog kibbles. Why? Because we have become so accustomed to fat, sugar, and salt as the major taste components of our food.

There are thousands of food-related issues that concern all of us, from taste to calories. However, two consequences of diet stand out: health and weight (not necessarily in that order). These are interrelated, though perhaps not as directly as it might seem. I will deal with them separately.

Diet and Weight

Being overweight may not be as unhealthy as some think. It is not actually a direct risk factor for developing heart disease or experiencing sudden death. By itself, it won't shorten your life. It does, however, predispose an individual toward such risk factors as hypertension, hypercholesterolemia, and diabetes. Over the years, we have concluded that excess weight is bad for us because in most cases, it is accompanied—or even in part caused—by a sedentary lifestyle that allows the body to deteriorate while it increases in size. Then, too, we've been conditioned to see excess weight as physically unattractive. The next step to regarding obesity as unhealthy is to be too short.

The fact is that there is little evidence to indicate that excess weight, all by itself, is seriously bad for you—the exception being, of course, cases of such extreme obesity where the heart simply can't handle the load. Even a relatively high cholesterol count can be mitigated by a favorable high-density to low-density lipid ratio (the legendary good fat/bad fat mix), which can frequently be achieved by exercise. Body types also differ, and what's too much weight for one person is not for someone else. We can't judge everyone on the same scale. Now, if only someone would break the news to Hollywood and Madison Avenue....

The real issue in weight gain is psychological. Gaining weight can make you feel bad about yourself—just another stressor you don't need. Those of us who have worked in diet clinics can recognize and appreciate the low self-esteem of individuals there for help losing weight.

Nonetheless, it comes as no surprise that there is far too much obesity in American culture. With the strong association our culture makes between inactivity and luxury, along with some of the food values we treasure, the only thing that's truly surprising is that more people aren't overweight. Have you heard how hard it is for American tourists to fit into Japanese bus seats?

Is weight gain an inevitable part of the aging process? We do tend to gain fat and lose muscle mass as we age, yet such a change need not be inevitable. Midlife weight gain comes less from physiological factors (though our nutritional needs do change) than from living an increasingly sedentary existence. In short, we tend to sit on our butts more.

When was the last time you played nine hard innings, four nonstop quarters, or three sets? Or when did you last try to keep up with a four year old for a day? Because of desk jobs and an inevitable, if not incremental, loss of muscle strength—a vicious circle—we ultimately end up just not as active as we once were.

For many, the most common reaction to weight gain is to go on a crash diet or start some weird eating program. These we might try to do instead of owning up to the fact that we are getting older and just need to learn to eat more judiciously.

When most people decide to diet, they approach it all wrong by trying to attack the problem episodically rather than as a long-term endeavor. That is to say, they figure that they'll diet this week so that maybe they can go back to their old, bad habits next week—sort of like gathering a line of credit in dietary virtue.

Of course, it doesn't work. It may take a few pounds off temporarily, but the weight comes right back once the diet ends. What's needed is a sane, doable switch to reasonable eating habits that can last the rest of your lifetime. Ideally, these habits should include an intelligent mixture of the appropriate food groups with appropriate physical activity.

Such a two-pronged attack is the best course. If we stay active in the first place, most of our dietary problems will take care of themselves. Combined with a sensible diet, good honest activity can go a long way toward keeping us at our perfect weight.

Many people wanting to lose weight seek a magic bullet in the form of an herb or prescription drug. From the *Encyclopedia of Natural Medicine,* we learn that authors Michael Murray, N.D., and Joseph Pizzorna, N.D., refer to Ma huang (ephedra sinica), cola nut (cola nitida), and green tea (Camellia sinensis) as "isolated plant stimulants which promote fat breakdown. Although many stimulants [like these] are routinely abused in our current society, the use of plants as stimulants has a long history of use by the majority of cultures worldwide."

It is interesting to note that these three substances can be found easily at your local drugstore. Ephedra contains ephedrine and related alkaloids. The two others, Cola nitida and Camellia sinensis, are chock-full of caffeine, theophylline, and other methyl xanthines known to speed up your motor, as it were. Using any of these, the authors insist, can assist any man significantly overweight in his personal quest for thinness. Certainly, researchers have isolated and quantified the efficacy of these specific ingredients. It may be another matter, however, to "extrapolate" such data to a crude herb or extract.

Ephedrine alone, especially with one of the methyl xanthines like caffeine or theophylline in experimental animal studies, jacks up the metabolic rate of your adipose (fat) tissue. Human studies corroborate that it is the combination of these herbs that will increase the metabolic rate in anyone who is obese.

Now for some controversy. A researcher named Jason Lazarou, in the April 15, 1998, issue of the *Journal of the American Medical Association,* describes Adverse Drug Reactions (ADR). He emphasized that ADRs are all too frequent and, in fact, are between the fourth and sixth leading cause of death. Ironically, in hospitals the majority of ADR problems are "due to inadequate monitoring or therapies and doses." The numbers are frightening: "In 1994 in the United States, 106,000 hospitalized patients died from an ADR." So the challenge remains for the discerning clinician just how significant the risks of herbs such as Ma huang (ephedra) really are.

Studies show that Ma huang may indeed increase the heart rate of some volunteers who have normal blood pressure. But so does a sauna. All in all, Ma huang had variable effects on blood pressure. Interestingly, a random analysis of this traditional Chinese herb using gas chromatography failed to show any nasty synthetic isomers, such as synthetic Ephedra alkaloids.

We all became gun shy after the weight-loss drugs Redux (dexfenfluramine) and Pondimin (fenfluramine), part of the popular fen-phen combination, were unceremoniously removed from the market in 1997. Even so, there are a lot of entrepreneurs anxious to offer a "natural" replacement for these products. According to the January–February 1998 issue of *FDA Consumer,* the range of recorded complications have included "high blood pressure and headaches to heart attacks and [even] death." Such warnings certainly ring familiar with what Lazarou chronicled as all-too-frequent ADRs from properly approved FDA drugs. Let us not ignore some 1,500 documented cases including 38 deaths from a rare blood disorder from another fen-phen product, 5-hydroxy tryptophan, closely related to L-tryptophan.

The take-home advice from this allopathic physician is that you run about as great a chance of running into a problem taking an ephedrine product as, let's say, popping amoxicillin for bronchitis or the codeine derivative in Vicoden. Make sure that you review your natural remedies with a naturopath or, at least, the purveyor where you buy the potion of your choice. I wouldn't take a drop myself until I reviewed the drug with Dr. David Lu, a third generation Chinese herbalist and acupuncturist now in Minneapolis who knows alternative pharmaceuticals the way I know western synthetic drugs. Knowing as much as possible can ensure smooth sailing without any unwanted drug reactions.

Diet and Fat

Most desperation dieters do a couple of very predictable things. First, they radically reduce the quantity of food they eat. Second, they go on a crusade to eliminate fat. Although cutting down on the fat may be good if kept within rational bounds, cutting it out entirely is not only unnecessary but potentially unsafe, especially among children (don't forget essential fatty acids).

We certainly don't require nearly as much fat—certainly not as much as the average American consumes—but we do need to eat a basic minimum of the so-called essential fats required to maintain cell or nerve membrane synthesis. Cholesterol, believe it or not, is important for the production of steroids, which are so important in the manufacturing of hormones. Fats (including cholesterol) are components of the myelin that is a critical part of your nerve sheaths. Lipids (fats) are therefore essential to the health of your brain and the senses linking you to the outside world. That devil cholesterol also turns out to be an important part of the structure of your cell walls as well as a major component of your sex hormones.

Nevertheless, fat and cholesterol are prime suspects for causing heart disease. Left unmetabolized, cholesterol will deposit itself all over the circulatory system, especially in the coronary arteries that service your heart. That, as we all know, can be bad, very bad.

Our bodies can also manufacture cholesterol. Eating all those nice new cholesterol-free foods can be great, but not all that useful if you happen to be someone who just happens to produce too much cholesterol. Uncontrolled consumption of other fats, protein, or carbohydrate in large quantities still leads to obesity, which, although not as serious a direct cardiac risk factor, may predispose you to other cardiac risk factors such as hypertension or diabetes.

A sedentary body can be an invitation to heart disease. An active, fit body should be able to store fats as high-density lipids, which are like paratroopers at the door, helmets on, clipped in, and ready to jump into the bloodstream not only as nutrients to reinforce tired active muscles but also as protection against lipid plaques, the silent killers of myocardial infarction or stroke.

We are conditioned by habit, heredity, culture, and even fate to like fats. If you cut out all the oil (fat) that titillates hungry taste buds, your food just doesn't seem to slide down as smoothly. You could run the risk of becoming one of those ascetics who eat to live rather than live to eat. Reducing excess animal fat, simple sugars, and protein (the surplus of which is converted to fat) is one way to control so-called android obesity experienced by guys in their forties with those characteristic love handles around their waists. (The complement in women is gynoid obesity, or cellulite deposits around their hips and thighs, also known not so fondly as saddlebags.)

Historically, fat has played a major role in human survival. Fat gave us endurance in cold climates and enabled us to survive during those long periods when a daily meal was not a foregone conclusion. Once our bodies ran out of carbohydrate energy in the form of easily metabolized glycogen stored in the muscles or liver, we needed a secondary source of energy—the fat by which our bodies store nutrients.

The recent experience of polar explorers tells the tale. Minnesota's Will Steger, in his 1986 dogsled dash to the North Pole, virtually survived on fats. He poured butter on his morning oatmeal and ate pemmican (80 percent animal fat or better) as the major component of the rest of his diet. He crammed in 7,000 calories a day eating this killer diet, lost weight, and never had a cholesterol problem. His secret? Grinding, exhausting work, day after day, in a cold setting that had his metabolism burning on high just to stay warm. This is a close parallel to camping next to a polar ice cap and hunting for a living with spears and sharpened rocks.

There is also evidence gathered from the native Inuit of northern Canada suggesting that despite a diet that is largely red meat and muktuk (whale blubber), they suffer from very little heart disease. Interestingly, their diet also includes lots of fish, high in alpha epicoacanthoic acid, which is extremely effective in metabolizing fats.

Actually, there are far simpler methods than surviving the great North in order to accomplish fat reduction. A British study cited in *Food & Wine Magazine* suggests that taking a walk before eating can reduce the effects of eating fats. The study, conducted at Loughborough University, found that subjects who ate a high-fat meal after a 2-hour walk had a 31 percent lower triglyceride level than those who ate the same meal and after no exercise. The researchers also concluded that exercise after eating also has beneficial effects.

Diet and Culture

Rice and beans are perhaps the most common foodstuffs on our planet and are popular from Mexico City to Kuala Lumpur and at every point in between. Even though they sound rather ordinary, they are yet another proof that nature is an intelligent provider. For between them they offer complete protein, lots of fiber and vitamins, a paucity of fat, and plenty of carbohydrates.

But while all this healthy eating is going on down in the huts, up in the hacienda, the master is eating rich cuts of beef and pork with lots of butter sauces, eggs, and refined sugar—the works. So what happens when the proletariat become affluent, as they have in Europe and North America? Do they keep their former diet? Heck, no! They always envied the landed gentry for their luxuries, so now they just dig into the fats and sugars with gusto. Their former foods—the funky, found-it-under-a-rock stuff they used to have to eat for protein—may still be snails, sweetmeats, frog legs, and other such gourmet items. Only now they're covered with cream and butter sauces.

Yes, indeed, affluence has a huge influence on diet… but not all for the better!

Fat and Health

How much body fat is OK? How do we know? We've learned that actuarial tables allow for an increase in weight as we age. But because muscle is denser than fat, any weight gain could hide an even greater increase in body fat that many of us (and our hearts) end up lugging around.

Should you aim to maintain the weight you had at the end of high school, or should you accept an extra 10 pounds? Your high school weight (assuming you were fit then) is a reasonable target from a health standpoint but may not always be realistic. You didn't sit at a desk all day back then—not voluntarily, at least. These 10 extra pounds are not too dire, but you should remember that they are a realistic compromise, and not necessarily the ideal.

There are several methods for determining just how much of us is fat. The three most common techniques are caliper, electrical impedance, and underwater immersion. Consensus is that although immersion may be the most accurate, the complex gear required to perform this scientific form of baptism can be prohibitively expensive. Not only must there be a large enough tank into which subjects are lowered, but also lung volume must be analyzed inside an airtight container to subtract from the water displaced in the dunk tank.

With significant practice (hundreds of measurements, actually), the caliper method has gained a reputation for ballpark accuracy. Plus, the price is right—only one experienced technician is needed. Impedance has generally received mixed reviews. It has been judged fine for those in the middle of the pack, but for others—that is, the massively obese or those who are all skin and bones—it is not as reliable. In terms of screening a fairly athletic population, impedance can be fast and accurate enough and can eliminate a lot of messy calculations. On the whole, the average health club is probably better off with the simplicity and reproducibility of impedance techniques despite their limitations. In a sense, this method is more reproducible and less dependent on an experienced technician.

For the general population, a body fat composition of 7 to 13 percent for men in their forties, less than 14 percent for men in their fifties, and less than 15 percent for men in their sixties fits into the "excellent" category. But according to University of Minnesota cardiologist and epidemiologist Art Leon, MD, these low numbers may be unrealistic and even unhealthy for some people. According to Leon, an average fat composition is more like 17 to 23 percent for men in their forties, 18 to 24 percent for men in their fifties, and 19 to 25 percent for men in their sixties.

Just to keep any of you from becoming smug, elite male marathon runners have an average body fat range of 4 to 7 percent. Elite female runners can have 12 to 17 percent body fat. Some women may carry even less, but as their body fat drops, they risk getting sick or developing menstrual irregularity.

Though men are not usually known to become anorexic, it is possible to overexercise and undereat to the point of risking injury. For example, if you're participating in cold-weather activities, you should take care not to drop below 4 percent body fat. You have a much greater chance of developing hypothermia or becoming otherwise sick at these lower levels.

As I've mentioned before, all fat isn't bad, and some is necessary. But there is still an overabundance of saturated fats in the American diet. Saturated fats, found in meat and dairy products, are generally hard at room temperature. This is also true for naturally hard vegetable oils such as coconut or palm oils, which until recently were often present in such innocuous products as nondairy creamers. These oils should be minimized. If you can, replace them with relatively unsaturated fats such as olive, canola, or safflower oils. This is where it pays to read the product labels.

Also important is the time of day you eat, as well as the quantity and composition of your daily 4,000 calories. Sure, the old American standby of bacon, eggs, hash browns, and toast saturated with melted butter certainly means starting the day with plenty of calories to last until the 10:00 A.M. midmorning break. But this meal was devised to send farmers off to a hard day of labor in the fields. In other words, they would work it all off.

But in the latter half of the twentieth century (and the beginning of the twenty-first), our jobs are different and involve more sitting on your butt than tilling the field. Thus it makes more sense to replace most of that breakfast fat and protein with the complex carbohydrates found in a steaming bowl of high-fiber oatmeal, whole-grain pancakes, or raisin-cinnamon bagels with low-fat cream cheese, and washed down with lots of unsweetened orange juice.

THE FRENCH PARADOX

As we become more knowledgeable of what our male brethren in other countries are eating and drinking, we may get an idea of types of diets that seem to work. We know damn well that our high-fat, high-meat intake in the United States isn't good for the heart. But what is? Now researchers are studying how the French can consume all those rich cheeses and luscious desserts (not to mention all their wonderful wines) and yet have a heart failure rate much lower than that of their American counterparts. The results seem to point to three major dietary differences.

1. The French eat more fresh vegetables and fruits. Instead of "Le Beeg Mac," they might opt for a plate of greens as crudités (raw vegetables), marinated beans, or ratatouille, a tasty blend of tomatoes, eggplants, and onions stirred in olive oil and garlic and seasoned with fresh herbs.

2. The French eat less red meat but more fermented dairy products. It's well known that the fats in red meats and dairy products, if taken too often, can lead to cholesterol problems and hardening of the arteries. But recent studies in France have indicated that when dairy fats go through fermentation, as in the process of converting milk or cream into cheese, they bind up with calcium and become much more difficult for the stomach to absorb. In other words, the fats in cheese move right through the system and, voilà, are eliminated. Fats found in milk, cream, and ice cream, on the other hand, are much more easily absorbed.

3. The French drink more wine, particularly red wine. The evidence here is still coming in, but it seems to indicate that drinking wine in moderation—one to three glasses a day—inhibits the production of cholesterol in the body, and that red wine is more effective at this than white. And we all know, of course, that the French drink ample quantities of wine.

Nutrition and Health

So what's the latest wisdom in nutrition? Oat bran? Cod liver oil? Broccoli? Just say no?

Nutrition has lately been a source of some wonderful pop culture as well as plenty of misinformation. It seems that every time the TV news runs into a slow news day, you can be treated to the latest in miracle diets to lengthen your life or improve your mood. The question is, how much of this stuff is real?

You should know that there may be a lot of truth in these ideas. The right diet could lower your cholesterol, your blood pressure, and your risk for certain cancers.

Fiber

Fiber has been a dietary holy grail for over a decade now. According to sports nutritionist Ellen Coleman, RD, of the Sports Clinic, Riverside, California, "a high fiber diet may also help to prevent diverticular disease, colon cancer, diabetes, and cardiovascular disease."

Actually, the way fiber works is very prosaic—more than anything, further evidence that nature, in its basic form, provides well for all of us. Humankind has known for centuries that roughage "keeps you regular." Fiber contains structural plant material that supplies bulk to your system. The more vegetables, grains, and legumes you consume, the more bulk can pass through your system. Fiber is not some miracle chemical; it merely makes your alimentary canal work more efficiently. By adding volume to your stool, fiber helps your body's waste travel through the colon quicker. This means that toxins and carcinogens are removed at a faster rate. The net effect is that fiber seems to keep us "cleaner" inside.

Your fiber intake should be about 25 to 50 grams a day. Foods such as beans, corn, peas, oat bran, prunes, blueberries, and raisins are fiber factories. Eat them if you want to be healthy.

Vitamins

Fortunately, as we age, we normally get all the vitamins we need from a balanced diet. Yet should you take some vitamins, such as the so-called antioxidants—vitamins E, A, and C, plus beta-carotene, selenium, and the food additives BHA and BHT—in larger quantities? The jury still seems to be out, but evidence does suggest that antioxidants are beneficial. These vitamins combat free radicals in the body—rogue oxygen ions that go around creating havoc with otherwise stable, happy, and healthy complex molecules. The theoretical outcome is that among other benefits, the body's natural process of aging will be slowed.

Eating fruits and vegetables rich in vitamin C and beta-carotene such as broccoli, brussels sprouts, or cauliflower may reduce your risk from certain types of cancer, especially colon cancer. We don't always know why, but statistics just don't seem to lie. Possibly the anticancer effect has something to do with a combination of nutrients and fiber.

By all means, try to keep the vitamin content in the food you eat as high as possible. Raw food, of course, has the most vitamins, but cooking food carefully can still be okay. Don't cook your veggies to death. If you must have them softened and warm, try steaming or stir-frying them in order to retain their vitamins.

This has triggered something of a mini-revolution in Western cuisine. It's said that you should never accept a dinner invitation from an Englishman more than two weeks in advance, because when the invitations go out, they put the vegetables on to boil. These days, we take our example of how to cook our vegetables from the Asians—heated just enough to let the herbs and spices enhance the flavor, but not enough to make them limp and void of nutritional value.

Most vitamin supplements probably can't hurt, although Ellen Coleman contends that because the average endurance athlete eats like a pig anyway just to maintain ideal body weight, he or she is unlikely to become deficient in vitamins and minerals. Ideally, eating plenty of fresh fruits and vegetables can replenish vital vitamin stores while giving you all the fiber you ever wanted.

Dairy

The ideal amount you should eat from the dairy group (milk, yogurt, and cheese) is 2 to 3 servings per day. Again, don't overdo it. Is it a myth that consuming too much dairy will make you produce too much mucous? Dr. Benjamin Spock and friends did not gain favored-citizen status in Wisconsin or Vermont (where as little as 30 years ago there were more cows than people) by criticizing children drinking too much milk. Skim milk is an excellent source of protein and carbohydrate and is negligible in fat. There are also fat-free whole-milk alternatives now available that may taste even better than previously available nonfat products.

Keep in mind that as you become an adult, your ability to process dairy products may diminish. Part of this is a function of the natural aging system. Another part is simply that you begin consuming fewer dairy products, particularly milk and ice cream—two very popular kid foods. And as you consume less, your system may slowly lose its ability to process them. Physicians attribute this difficulty to a lactase deficiency, the enzyme that digests mill products (lactose) in your gut.

Some nutritionists feel that dairy products do more harm than good for the aging male body by supplying little nutritional value but lots of fat (unless your thing happens to be skim milk), as well as causing flatulence, stomach upset, excess mucous production, and even allergies.

The bottom line is that if you've consumed dairy products all your life, there's no reason to stop now unless you feel they're giving you problems. But by all means, minimize the high-fat stuff: Choose skim or 1 percent milk and cottage cheese, be careful with the half-and-half (I confess I like it in my coffee, although there is a perfectly palatable nonfat alternative), and by all means avoid full-fat chocolate sundaes. (As for cheeses, see "The French Paradox" on page 148.)

Iron

One advantage of being male is that you shouldn't have to worry too much whether you are getting enough iron. Because you don't menstruate, almost all the iron from red cells breaking apart every 120 days gets recycled into your iron pool via your liver and spleen. But even in the male, there are insensible losses through sweating or simply by passing stool. Recent studies confirm a significant blood loss that bypasses this recycling loop in the endurance athlete who is vigorously training, resulting in runner's or athlete's anemia.

Researchers from Minneapolis and the Mayo Clinic have used a technique called the HemaQuant method to quantify blood loss among athletes after a marathon. They have discovered appreciable losses among two groups: those who were less well trained and those who were younger. Any male 40 and over who's doing significant physical activity should check his blood count yearly. A low hemoglobin and especially low indices (the size and concentration of hemoglobin in the red cells, called "mean corpuscular volume") should alert your physician to obtain iron levels and a serum ferritin. A low serum iron—the saturation of the transferring stores that hold the iron—means there is plenty of room within your iron stores for more iron, and a workup looking for a hidden loss of blood from somewhere in your system becomes mandatory.

The red herring is "foot-strike" hemolysis (the runner's anemia already mentioned) or some other cause of blood loss due to, for example, hemolysis of red cells within the kidney itself. Either of these can contribute to an athlete's anemia. This can be especially true if you happen to be a vegetarian. The sad truth for noncarnivores is that the non-heme (blood) iron such as that found in spinach or iron pills, for example, isn't efficiently absorbed from your ileum the way iron from red meat is.

WHERE WE GO WRONG

We need to achieve good nutrition without excess consumption. The trouble is that our desires and lifestyles conspire to get in the way. For example, in the haste to get out the door in the morning, breakfast often becomes secondary to time clocks, work deadlines, and getting kids off to school. And though a bowl of cereal is better than a slab of toast, and a slab of toast is better than nothing, neither may supply enough protein or unsaturated fat to get you to your midmorning snack.

If you happen to be a construction worker who works outside in the elements all day, you should toss down plenty of nonfat yogurt as well as oatmeal or pancakes. They're making turkey bacon now, in case you're hopelessly hooked on this popular bit of gustatory Americana—but try to get it without the nitrates, which have been implicated as an increased cancer risk. Another booster is some whole wheat toast or a bagel with thinly sliced goat cheese, negligible in saturated fat.

The Components of a Proper Diet

A balanced diet is on the one hand very complex—the body requires a huge number of nutrients, some in very small quantities and others in greater quantity. As I've mentioned earlier, human beings can get a balanced diet from simple combinations, for example, of rice and beans, fresh fruits and vegetables, and a small amount of meat, eggs, or dairy products. Let's look at the basic components, illustrated by the Food Guide Pyramid:

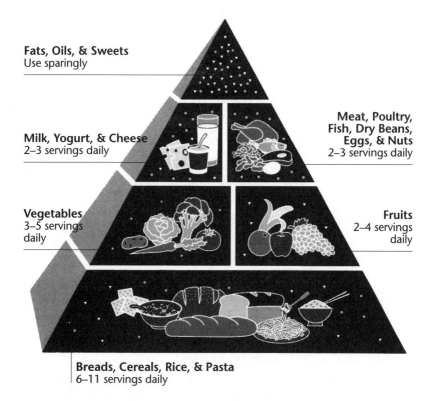

Fats, Oils, & Sweets
Use sparingly

Milk, Yogurt, & Cheese
2–3 servings daily

**Meat, Poultry,
Fish, Dry Beans,
Eggs, & Nuts**
2–3 servings daily

Vegetables
3–5 servings
daily

Fruits
2–4 servings
daily

Breads, Cereals, Rice, & Pasta
6–11 servings daily

Carbohydrates

Carbohydrates form the base of the pyramid, and they include breads, cereals, rice, and pasta. Eat 6 to 11 servings from the grain group each day. Carbohydrates are a most useful food group, which is why dietary experts are continually revising upward their suggestions of the percentage of carbohydrates in a good diet. It is not excessive to consume 60 percent of your regular diet as "carbs." This is especially true if you happen to be regularly athletic and need to replenish your glycogen stores often.

Carbs are useful largely because they can be easily metabolized in the body for energy. If consumed in moderation, they are far more beneficial than fats, which like to glom onto your stomach, your butt, or, worse yet, your coronary arteries. Carbohydrates are stored in your muscles, liver, or blood in the form of glycogen, a complex sugar that can be quickly put to use by your muscles as glucose when you need it. You are also capable of manufacturing glucose (gluconeogenesis) from protein when your glycogen stores become depleted, but this means the body feeding on the stuff that's supposed to be building you up—sort of like internal cannibalization.

Endurance athletes are famous for "carbo loading" on the day or sometimes the week before a big endurance event. By pigging out at a spaghetti feed, they try to load as much glycogen into their muscle tissues as possible. Some swear by plenty of beer to wash it down. The experts are skeptical. Their ultimate goal is to put all the fuel they have stored in their liver or muscles to use in the race the next day.

Some athletes have learned how to supercharge their glycogen stores by depleting them for a week while they eat just fat and protein. Take my word, this diet is lethal. Recall that the brain thrives on glucose, and there isn't a lot of that around during a depletion phase of carbo loading. The key factor is that the central nervous system depends on carbohydrates almost completely for its nutrition until it can shift over to fat metabolism. The more civilized approach to preparing for an endurance event such as a marathon is simply to increase your daily carbohydrate intake starting 1 week before the event and skip the uncomfortable depletion phase. In other words, eat like a pig, but eat wisely.

Diet programs are emphasizing proteins in an effort to supplement the dieter who may tend toward tissue breakdown to compensate for marked calorie restriction. There are commercial and natural medications available that can make this otherwise torturous regimen feasible. If you have too much paranoia of idiopathic pulmonary hypertension from this combination, consider "natural" alternatives, such as Ma huang, very active in ephedra and a natural stimulant.

Ever hear of "hitting the wall?" Some athletes call it "bonking." This is when you're running a race and you suddenly imagine a large woolly bear jumping out of the woods to grab you. Or something like that. Your race as you hoped to know it is now over, and you have entered a basic and painful survival mode. Your biggest challenge from this point until the finish line is to avoid tripping over your tongue.

Here's what happens: As you run, you begin to use up all the glycogen in your tissues. When the glucose levels get low enough, your body goes into its second line of defense and switches over to less efficient fat metabolism. At this point, unless you get some nutrition quickly to refurbish your stores with carbohydrates, you've had it, and your race is over.

As we all know, there is a downside to eating too much carbohydrate. The excess caloric intake can be stored as fat. Too much sugar in the body (which carbohydrates become after ingestion) may also lead to obesity, diabetes, or even coronary artery disease. High lipid (fat) levels irrefutably lead to clogged coronaries.

What about the old advice to eat a candy bar before exercising? Forget it. This superstition has gone out of favor on the theory that this onslaught of simple sugars will trigger a flood of insulin to be released into your body, soon tossing you into a low-sugar wasteland by swiftly using up all your available carbohydrate stores. In other words, the insulin surge you precipitated has eaten up not only the candy bar but all your glycogen stores as well. Talk about hitting the wall. So don't go pounding down a regular Coke and then take off running. If you need that caffeine-sugar hit, wait till you're past the halfway mark, preferably until three-quarter way through an endurance race. Beverages such as Gatorade and Quench, which are high in polycose (an easily absorbable sugar) and electrolytes, are another challenging topic. Such fluids of the correct concentration and temperature can help sustain your glucose levels and keep you from plummeting into that never-never land of anaerobic metabolism when you shift into less efficient fat metabolism. Even small amounts of glucose, however, can slow absorption of water from the stomach. Meanwhile, studies show that glucose polymers, unlike plain sugar solutions, in fact increase the movement of water from the stomach.

Carbs thus play an important role in keeping your body going and in good shape. However, like almost everything you put in your body, there is a right amount (use in moderation, dependent upon body type and exercise level) and a right type (prefer complex over simple). Use your head, and your body will follow.

Protein

OK, back to high school. Remember health class? The nutrition unit that was entitled "Protein: Building Block of a Healthy Body"? Well, protein is still important, especially if you want enough muscle mass to get you out of bed in the morning. The real question is *how* you get your protein, not whether protein per se is good for you.

Protein intake in North America has, up until a few years ago, increasingly come from red meat, and with it has come a high content of saturated fats. Most of the world, however, gets its protein from vegetable sources such as the aforementioned universal proletarian fare of beans and rice.

Which is the best way? Fortunately, in our advanced society, most of us have a choice of how we may consume the 2 to 3 daily servings of protein, whether it be red meat, white meat, fish, dairy, whole grains, or legumes. Unfortunately, our tastes and our society dictate that we don't always choose what's best for us.

The solution, unless you're going totally vegetarian, is to compromise. In other words, buy meat but make sure it's lean. Limit your consumption by including red meats in fewer meals or, as Asian cultures prefer, in smaller quantities. This is one of the obvious advantages of stir-fried foods. Asian foods tend to be low in fat, high in quickly cooked fresh vegetables, high in natural vitamins, and perfect with a vat of steaming rice (brown, white, wild, Basmati)—unbeatable for an evening meal, both in flavor and nutrition. Try your pastas without meatballs. Instead, use cheeses (Parmesan or other), chopped nut meats, shrimp, or veggies stirred into your sauce.

Eat more broiled fish and skinless chicken. Be wary of that other white meat, pork, but be assured that it is still leaner than red meat. Pork's charm is that it goes a long way in small quantities. Where you'd eat a pound of beef in a slab, you'd need only a few ounces of pork with vegetables in a delicate, yet tasty light soy sauce. Pork, however, especially in its more baroque permutations such as sausage, can be high in fat, which is added for taste. Enjoy it but don't overdo it.

In the dairy department, much of what you can now buy is nonfat. Particularly appealing is nonfat or low-fat sour cream for slathering on a yam or baked potato. The sour cream offers protein and calcium, and the yam supplies vitamins (particularly A), fiber, and complex carbohydrate. A creatively prepared baked potato makes a delightful evening meal, smothered in healthy tidbits like natural cheeses, nonfat sour cream, scallions, and even salsa. And don't forget to eat the skin—it's high in fiber.

Eggs can also be good for you, especially if the cholesterol has been removed. They are as high in biologically perfect protein as any food you are going to find.

It's just plain challenging being a vegophile. First off, we're conditioned to eat meat in a society that gobbles burgers, ribs, and steak by the boxcar. Further, some folks are still threatened by anyone who doesn't eat meat and often perceive vegetarians as weird or subversive (subversive maybe, low blood pressure, absolutely; lower LDL, total cholesterol, usually).

If you're vegetarian, you must get what protein you need from dried beans (legumes) and legume derivatives such as tofu, eggs (or egg substitutes), and nuts—though the latter carry the downside of high fat. For the vegetarian on the run, it is often difficult to create a complete protein. Their challenge is in combining the complementary amino acids from the three groups of the vegetable proteins correctly. In general, serving a whole grain (brown rice, cracked wheat, barley) with a legume (beans, peas, lentils, tofu) successfully combines complementary amino acids to build a complete protein mix. But this is not always easy when you're on the open road with three screaming kids who want to go to McDonald's for a Happy Meal. It's a simple fact that meat is still the easiest, most readily available, and complete source of protein we have in our modern society.

Though eating enough protein should not be a problem for most Americans, vegetarians should consciously monitor their iron intake to prevent iron deficiency anemia. Heme iron from red meats is absorbed so much better than from any nonmeat source. If you don't get enough heme iron, iron supplements might be useful.

For diehard vegetarians, all this extra effort is well worth it. Overall, they have lower body fat, lower blood pressure, and lower rates of heart disease, stroke, and bowel cancer. Not only do they live longer, but they often enjoy a healthier life than those who are predominantly carnivores.

Doing It Right: Designing a Diet for the Future

By now you should know that you don't have to blame yourself if your mouth waters every time you see a TV commercial featuring a juicy, tender steak sizzling over an open fire. Like Pavlov's dog, you've been conditioned to think that way. And, sorry to say, you might never quite get over it. I know of an over-40 Hollywood agent who was a vegetarian for 364 days of the year. On the 365th day he would go out for a steak. (I'm not sure what he did on leap years.) The last time I heard, he was no longer a vegetarian but instead had chosen a middle ground of basic healthy eating incorporating some meat from time to time.

Hunger is a triggered response, and the feeling doesn't go away until you satisfy it. You can learn to control or even eliminate your hunger pangs under certain circumstances. You have a great deal of latitude in how you respond to hunger. That is to say, you can control what you actually eat when you get hungry.

Regretfully, it may be a little late for dietary control to come easy. If you were brought up on Sugar Corn Pops and 19¢ hamburgers, it may be tough to make the change to a healthier diet. Yet this doesn't have to be the same for your kids. Despite the abundance of TV commercials selling caffeinated soda pop, high-fat fast foods, and high-sugar, low-fiber cereals to the youngest generation, you can counter the electronic mind-blitz with your own example of healthy eating and just plain common sense. Push fresh fruits and vegetables for snacks. Kids love bananas, oranges, apples, pears, grapes, carrots, and other finger foods for afternoon snacks. Special treats might include yogurt ice cream, ice pops, Jell-O or fruit with yogurt toppings, and low-fat multigrain cookies. In other words, don't get them used to the same sugar and fat diet you might be battling. In 30 years, you don't want your kids to be in the same position you're in now.

So how do you do it?

Snacking Between Meals

Even health food aficionados meet their downfall when it comes to those long empty periods between meals. Yet there are ways to remedy hunger urges in a positive way.

Snacking by itself is not bad. In fact, experts suggest that the three-meal-a-day system is not how we were meant to eat anyway. Back in the hunter-gatherer days there was about a 3-second delay between downing our fallen prey and popping it into our mouths. Even back at the cave, it's unlikely that we sat down at regular intervals, said grace, and chowed down with our napkins on our laps. We ate as we could, when we could, and usually were plenty hungry.

There are interesting analogies within the animal kingdom. The Siberian tiger will sleep during the hottest time of the day, awaken at 9:00

P.M., and begin browsing for his supper—a time when he will need the least amount of energy expenditure. Dolphins become playful after they have consumed a big school of fish and are satiated. It's true with animals and with people that diet and energy levels for play and work (exercise) are neatly intertwined with how full stomachs are.

Whereas the urge to snack often means hunger—an indication that the body is asking for nourishment—it might also mean that you're bored, tired, angry, happy, in love, out of love, nervous, lonely, or (toughest of all) trying to quit smoking. In other words, you must become aware of your reason for wanting that snack. Because hunger responds to a variety of cues, you have to be careful not to let your perceived oral needs get you into trouble. In other words, snack smart.

How? First, cut out the snacks when you're not truly hungry. In fact, try to cut out eating altogether when you really don't need to eat. That includes chips in front of the TV, stopping at the pub after work, and, of course, that late-night bowl of ice cream.

But when you're truly hungry, you do need to eat. Ads for candy bars have played to this for years. There are some great alternatives, though. Here are some ideas:

If you're possessed by a sweet tooth, don't forget fruit. Bananas contain plenty of potassium and contain only about 70 to 100 calories. If you must have something to crunch, check out dried bananas and pineapples. Apples also supply that satisfying crunch, provide vitamin A, and are tremendously refreshing. Oranges are another terrific snack and are high in vitamin C. Plus you can eat as many as you like.

If you're hankering for some grain-based carbs, try a slab of whole-wheat toast, skip the butter, and spread on a layer of all-fruit (unsweet-ened) jam or jelly. For a midmorning snack, try a container of nonfat yogurt; it's only around 100 calories.

Do you ever get into the midafternoon and start to run on empty? This is a common occurrence, once again caused by gaps in your intake. Take heart—you can fight midafternoon blahs any number of ways. Try microwave popcorn, nonfat frozen yogurt, fruit, or low-fat whole-grain cookies. Now that carrots are available in peeled bite-sized pieces, they've become even more accessible as a great snack. Not only do they supply lots of vitamin A, but they satisfy that need to crunch.

For a time, anyway, an enlightened airline or two offered Dr. Cookie, a healthy alternative to the usual peanuts that come with your in-flight bev-erage. And speaking of flying, sitting for long hours in the dry air of a jet cabin can deplete your level of hydration as well as your potassium stores. So drink several glasses of water before, during, and after your flight. Eat a banana and drink lots of OJ—it's always on the beverage cart—to keep you from getting excessively tired or weak with hypokalemia (low potassium).

Eating Between Snacks

I've said earlier that gone are the days when the fat-laden bacon-and-egg breakfast is considered a healthy way to start the day. Unless you're out there really working in the fields from sunup to sundown, your body can't make use of all that fat, protein, and salt. Similarly, sweet rolls and donuts—oh my, what a temptation and oh, what empty calories. How many times have you run out the door in the morning without time for breakfast, only to arrive at work and inhale the donuts that just happen to be there? Hey, it's tough to say no. But what helps is taking that extra 15 minutes in the morning for a bowl of raisin bran or granola, for half a grapefruit and a piece of whole-wheat toast, or for a bowl of yogurt with fresh blueberries or raspberries or sliced peaches on top. Not only will a real breakfast be good for you, but you will feel better, too.

We all know about the importance of breakfast. But don't let all the hype blind you to an equal need for a healthy lunch and dinner. Traditionally, in this country, lunch was the big meal of the day. In the Midwest, some folks still call the midday meal "dinner" and the evening meal "supper" (from the old days when it was often just soup).

For today's power lunch, try filling that big hole in your stomach with plenty of water, fruits, and the offerings of an inventive salad bar. Go easy on the pasta salads, especially if the chef has smothered virginal macaroni in gobs of mayonnaise, which is high in highly saturated fat. (In case you didn't know, mayonnaise is made from egg yolks—a cholesterol bugaboo—and vegetable oil. It tastes great but is not less filling.)

If you're eating out of a lunch box, consider bringing to work or to workouts fruit, veggie sticks (celery, carrots, broccoli, cauliflower), and sandwiches to inhale safely when you need to replenish glycogen stores. If you come prepared, you won't find yourself stuffing coins into the nearest snack machine in order to abate your craving hunger.

Now we're coming to the tough part—and the eventual downfall of even the most dedicated diet ranger—dinner and afterward. A glass or two of wine or beer are okay, but don't rely on them for the liquid your body needs. Alcohol (due to so-called antidiuretic hormone, ADH) can dehydrate your system, and as we all know, beer tends to leave the body as quickly as it enters. Make sure when you serve alcoholic beverages to have water readily available, both for yourself and for your guests. Don't like the taste of tap water? Serve the bottled stuff. In Europe, water is the first thing they bring to your table. In Italy they ask, *"Gassata o non gassata?"*—"Do you want your water with gas (sparkling) or without?" First they plop the appointed water bottle on the table, then they bring the wine.

As for selecting a supper, don't forget that your eyes are always bigger than your stomach. In a sense, this is why a midafternoon snack may be good. If you come to the table famished, you're either going to order a big meal (if you're in a restaurant) or load your plate with everything in sight (if it's a buffet or you're at home). Mothers have been long aware that you never go to the grocery store on an empty stomach—the bill could easily double.

The Scandinavians, well known for their generally healthy ways, provide a good example for a tasty, yet low-calorie supper. They like to serve light sandwiches called smørbrød, which are thin slices of bread topped with margarine or butter and slices of fish, vegetables, or meat.

Desserts are always tough, but you can top off your evening meal with a cup of Jell-O, a quarter of a melon, or a small ice cream sandwich. Remember that a second glass of wine replaces dessert; this is one of those instances where you shouldn't drink your wine and eat your cake, too.

A while ago I remember meeting the one and only member of the Mexican Cross Country Ski Team, Robert "El Toro" Alvarez. He told me that his nutrition counselor limited him to one beer a night, which was a tall order for 6'4" skier who at one time was the Hispanic representative for Miller Beer in Milwaukee. Ah, what we won't do for our sport!

Fluids to Drink Before, During, and After Exercise

The fluids we choose to put into our bodies before, during, and after exercise have been the subject of hot debate. Witness the proliferation of electrolyte replacement and sports drinks already on the market. This public hype has plenty of basis in fact, because fluid balance has a lot to do with health. After all, more than 80 percent of your body is water, and virtually everything else is floating around in it. Hydration is especially important when you're working out, something you should keep in mind whenever the weather is especially hot. Likewise, when you sweat, regardless of the temperature, insensible losses of moisture can be appreciable.

Ellen Coleman recommends that anyone, but especially older athletes, should drink adequate liquids to decrease the risk of heatstroke or simply to perform better during exercise. This is a far cry from the days when we were admonished to limit fluid intake to avoid stomach cramps and we popped salt tablets for replacement.

According to Coleman, adequate hydration means 14 to 20 ounces of a rapidly absorbed fluid such as water or one of the polycose sports drinks 10 to 15 minutes before exercise, and at least 3 to 6 ounces every 20 minutes while exercising. Increase the intake if it's especially hot or if you think you're sweating more than usual.

Two warnings: (1) You generally become dehydrated well before you feel thirsty, so it's important to drink on a schedule rather than when you feel the need; and (2) cold fluids are absorbed faster than warm fluids. If you're using electrolyte replacement or sports drinks, it's important to mix them correctly. Either too much concentration or too little can inhibit absorption or just make you sick.

Should you pick one of the polycose carbohydrate solutions, you will benefit from the enhanced absorption of water as well as almost immediate energy replacement. Especially in prolonged exercise, fatty acids become your main source of energy once your muscle, liver, and blood glycogen stores are depleted. That's where such drinks can fit into your exercise picture. They can help supplement the glucose stores in your body that have become depleted.

Some people advocate drinking coffee before a workout or the big event, hoping the caffeine will release more free fatty acids and save some of their glycogen stores until later. Such a plan is fine if you are accustomed to the possible speeding effect caffeine can have. A better rule is generally not to try anything new on the day of your race or of an extended workout: no new running shoes, no new skis, no new race drinks.

On a visit some years back to his Palmer Lake, Colorado, home, the "Stretchmeister," Bob Anderson, author of the book *Stretching*, proudly showed me a Camelback water bottle—an easy way to supply great quantities of water during a long workout or marathon. "Don't leave home without it," he says. With it, you can go out on the trail for hours while sucking on a seemingly endless reservoir of your favorite liquid. This can allow you to carry on almost indefinitely.

Let's simplify. Drink a pint or so a half hour before exercise and a couple of swallows (okay, 6 ounces) every 15 to 20 minutes throughout your workout. And don't forget to replenish your liquid stores after your workout either—that's water or juice, not coffee or beer.

If you're in doubt about your diet, make a 3-day food record and have it analyzed by a dietitian. One caveat, however: It's going to be an exercise in futility if you're not honest about what you're eating. The diet log should tell no lies.

The bottom line is that you should keep your cholesterol, triglyceride, and low-density lipoproteins (LDL) levels at low levels, and your high-density lipoproteins (HDL) in the mid- to high range. Look to keep general fat intake low and other food groups in ideal balance.

Loading Up the Carbs

Careful complements of naturally occurring added fats can spice up your menu, and you still can maintain a high (60 percent) carbohydrate content to your diet.

Instead of loading up the meatballs the next time you have spaghetti, try sautéing skinless chicken breast strips in a tablespoon or two of naturally unsaturated garlic-flavored virgin olive oil. You can also add protein by sprinkling on naturally low-fat Parmesan cheese, one of the healthy white cheeses. Another option could be light roasting a nut meat, such as walnuts.

Another taste treat may take a little getting used to, but it's very popular with more adventuresome diners. Try whipping together mounds of pasta flavored with sesame paste or peanut butter, soy sauce, honey, and a wee bit of hot chili paste. The Chinese (who invented this scrumptious dish) love it cold. Keep in mind, though, that nut pastes such as peanut or sesame can be extremely high in calories and fat, so don't overdo them.

Or create your own pesto with a handful of fresh basil minced together with crushed pine nuts (walnuts will do), crushed garlic, olive oil, and salt. Some folks add a modest amount of the "liquor" left over from cooking the pasta. It can be served hot or cold—the latter makes a wonderful summer treat. If you don't have the time or the basil—it has to be fresh; dried won't do—pre-prepared pesto can often be found in the refrigerator section of your supermarket. Just be sure to read the label to make sure someone hasn't altered the basic recipe too much in the manufacturing process.

In short, reconsider your dietary habits. Why, for example, does anyone need to add salted butter to fresh young corn to enhance its flavor? If you're desperate, try artificial butter "buds," squeeze-tube margarines, or margarine-butter blends—not half bad if you just can't imagine corn being any good without butter. If that's still too tough, at least choose unsalted butter. Half a victory is better than no victory at all.

Speaking of Salt

According to some experts, the average American consumes two to three times the recommended amount of sodium a day. Yikes! The reason for this is simple: We're brought up on the stuff. Salt is everywhere. It hides out in canned foods (watch out for soup), nuts and nut butters, cheeses, processed meats, snack foods, sauces and dressings (particularly soy sauce), pickles, frozen meals, fast food—you name it. It even arrives naturally in, for instance, celery. Sodium is a legendary cause of elevated blood pressure, and salt is what puts many of the elderly in heart failure from fluid overload and hypertension.

Is there a substitute? Yes. There are potassium-based salts, but you don't want to overdo them either. How about MSG? Monosodium glutamate (MSG), often found in Chinese cooking, has about the same deleterious effect on your blood pressure as sodium-based table salt. For some people, MSG is immediately dangerous because it makes them drowsy. In fact, I believe that MSG should carry a warning on the label against operating machinery or a motorized vehicle after consuming it.

The bottom line here again is to use salt sparingly. Okay, at first low-salt dishes will taste bland to you. But eventually you'll get used to tasting the other flavors in the foods that salt has masked or overpowered. In fact, once you establish a low-salt diet, you'll be put off by many of the high-salt foods you formerly adored.

By the way, if you love Chinese food but don't want all the salt and MSG, simply ask the kitchen when you order for low (or no) salt and no MSG. The chefs in any decent Chinese restaurant will happily oblige.

Hold the Lard

It took many years, but finally many (if not most) processed foods are no longer likely to contain such ubiquitous sources of saturated fats as palm and coconut oils, butter, cream, meat fat, and lard—the latter once being a sneaky component of everything from Ma's apple pie to refried beans to fast-food french fries. If you're not sure whether a particular food contains saturated fats, read the label. (In the case of fast-food restaurants, ask for the nutritional breakdown sheet.) As you do so, look at the ingredients list and the nutritional table. Also remember that fat contains roughly twice the calories as an identical amount of carbohydrate or protein, so even if it's *good* fat, you don't want to consume too much.

Fortunately, food labeling has come a long way since yesteryear. Current prudent recommendations call for no more than 300 milligrams of cholesterol (from saturated fat) daily. As I've said earlier, recommendations for fat content in a healthy diet vary, ranging from a high of 30 percent (which I believe is too high) to a low of 10 percent (difficult to attain, but certainly admirable—and in any case, not impossible to achieve).

OK, you want to measure your fat intake. So how do you figure what percentage of your total caloric intake is from fat? One pencil method is to multiply the grams of fat in a serving by nine and then divide the result by the number of calories in the serving. The resulting figure shows the percentage of caloric intake that is from fat.

Example: Doritos Cool Ranch Chips contain 7 grams of fat in a 140-calorie serving. That's 7 gm. × 9 = 63, divided by 140, which comes out to a grand total of 45 percent fat. Yipes!

Take Your Vitamins

Americans spend millions of dollars annually on vitamins. There are many reasons for this, ranging from a belief that vitamins can cure and prevent illness, raise energy levels, and increase longevity, to a more rational desire of simply wanting to balance and supplement nutrition.

As I've mentioned earlier, there are two types of vitamins. The fat-soluble ones, such as A, D, E, and K, are stored in the body. Then there are the water-soluble ones, such as C, thiamine, riboflavin, B_6, niacin, folacin,

B_{12}, biotin, and pantothenic acid. Generally, it doesn't hurt to take vitamin supplements as long as you don't overconsume them. In most cases, they're not so much harmful as expensive. And eating a balanced diet meets the vitamin requirements for most men over 40. But studies have shown that taking too much of a fat-soluble vitamin can lead to severe toxicity. Even water-soluble vitamins can lead to problems. For example, complications have been reported for "mega" (10 times or more) doses of the recommended daily allowance (RDA) for vitamins C, niacin, and B_6.

Nevertheless, plenty of reasons exist to supplement certain vitamins at certain times—for instance, iron supplements during exercise or as an adjunct to a strict vegetarian diet. My advice is to discount the more extravagant claims for vitamins and nutritional supplements. But if you take them intelligently, they probably won't hurt you and may help. But expect to produce some mighty expensive urine.

Eat to Live, or Live to Eat?

In our modern society, eating is no longer a matter of survival. And a great deal about how we eat is cultural. Have you ever visited a good Italian family? You could drop over on a moment's notice—even in the middle of the night—and within minutes they would feed you something. Meals are among the most common rituals on earth—witness the formal diplomatic dinners engaged in by virtually every government.

In this society, we are bombarded by temptations to eat. Too many of these are high in fat, cholesterol, sugar, and salt. Too few offer the requisite amount of balanced nutrition and fiber. I don't want to impart any more guilt (America's number one killer) on the head of any 40-plus-year-old man. That's counterproductive. So I'll simply quote the Yiddish saying, *"Zie gezunt"*—"do it with gusto"—but add, "Always read the labels."

SUGGESTED READINGS

Brandenberg, Jeff. *Food Smart.* Rodale Press, 1996. 170 pp.

Lamm, Steven, MD. *Thinner at Last.* Simon and Schuster, 1966.

Lappé, Frances Moore. *Diet for a Small Planet.* Ballentine Fawcett, 1971.

Manahan, William. *Eat for Health.* HJ Kramer, 1988.

Moreman, Terri. *Official U.S. Olympic Training Table Cookbook.* Kraft General Foods, 1992. 76 pp.

Ornish, Dean, MD. *Eat More, Weigh Less.* Harper, 1997.

Pritikin, Robert, MD. *The New Pritikin Program.* Pocket Body Health, 1997.

Stephen, George. *Fight Fat.* Rodale Press, 1995. 170 pp.

A good source for creating well-balanced vegetarian meals can be found in Frances Moore Lappé's *Diet for A Small Planet.*

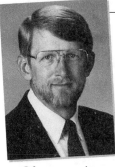

Jeff Bauer

Health Economist

Just entering his early fifties, Jeff Bauer looks every bit the part of his northern European ancestors—tall, stately, blond haired, blue eyed. In obvious good shape, he commands attention by his presence alone.

Of course, he could have gone the way of too many of his baby boomer colleagues—portly, slumped, looking older than his years. Yet Jeff has kept up with his early penchant for activity, though he has replaced the basketball games of his youth with running and the NordicTrack today.

As a health economist and consultant, Jeff spends approximately half his time either on airplanes or at some clinic or hospital many miles from his rural Colorado home. Anyone who has lived this lifestyle knows its drawbacks: long hours of sitting interspersed with airplane food, sometimes even longer drives in rental cars interspersed with road food. A real killer for the body. But Jeff takes time just before dinner almost every day to work out.

On the road, his preference is running. He'll aim for 2 to 3 miles or about 20 to 30 minutes. If he can't run, he'll swim at the hotel pool. At home he chooses the NordicTrack, which provides great all-around aerobic exercise. Again the aim is the 20- to 30-minute range.

Jeff couples his exercise with a healthy diet. Once an ardent meat eater, he now leans toward more fish and chicken for protein, whole grains and lots of veggies for substance and fiber. In fact, at home his family never has less than three raw vegetables on the table at each meal—during the summer and fall, almost all of it from their own garden. "We rarely cook veggies anymore," he says. "In fact, when I'm served cooked vegetables in restaurants, they taste odd." Agreeing with many nutritionists, he feels that cooking takes away too much of the good stuff that veggies offer.

Another advocacy of Jeff's is drinking plenty of water, something that's especially important for frequent flyers. As much as that cocktail is enticing, it wreaks havoc on the system when coupled with the thin, dry air of an airplane cabin. Though Jeff doesn't drink cocktails, he enjoys a glass or two of wine with his in-flight meals, followed (of course) by lots of water.

And speaking of wine, it is also part of Jeff's daily regimen. Though a native of the American West, the time he's spent in Europe has given him an indelible appreciation of fine wine and fine food. Though he likes whites, he prefers hearty California Zinfandels or Sangioveses, Spanish Riojas, French Côtes du Rhônes, or more ethereal Bordeaux.

profile

All in all, the Jeff Bauer theory for living well over 40 can be summarized fairly simply:

1. Exercise regularly, about 20 to 30 minutes a day.

2. Keep the fat intake down. Choose fish and chicken over red meats. (Jeff advocates oven grilling over outdoor barbecues to cut down the exposure to carcinogens from the charcoal fire.)

3. Eat lots of whole grains: granolas, oatmeal, whole-grain muffins and breads, for example.

4. Eat plenty of veggies; raw is preferred.

5. Drink lots of water.

6. Enjoy a bit of wine with your evening meal. (Recent evidence suggests that wine in moderation is beneficial to the cardiovascular system.)

Looking at Jeff and seeing his boundless energy is proof enough that his system works!

Chapter 10

Ways to Avoid Going Out of Your Mind

■ The Life Review and Other Tricks

> Age is not a particularly interesting subject. Anyone can get old. All you have to do is live long enough.
>
> Groucho Marx, *Groucho and Me*

The midlife passage has such a variety of negative effects on the male psyche that it has become a long-standing joke. You know—the one about the 45 year old who buys a toupee and a sports car, ditches his wife of 20 years, and starts wearing several large gold chains at a time.

But it's no joking matter. Midlife can be very stressful. The experience can be frightening at best, torturous at worst.

I've dealt with the whys of middle age in earlier chapters. Although there are a number of themes and problems common to all men, the stress you feel ends up being very real... and all your own. The particular mix of stress, anxiety, and life events that affects your feelings may be similar to those of other men, but they're never exactly the same.

So how do *you* feel about the 40th milestone?

If the stresses on your middle-aged psyche are unique, so too are the steps you can take to deal with them. You can adjust your own perceptions. The best way to reduce your stress may be to deal constructively with your feelings. In this chapter, I will discuss strategies for coming to terms with such stressors, and by so doing, help you discover ways of eliminating them.

One of the cardinal points to remember is that certain stress points are beyond your control. For example, if your boss happens to be a jerk, you'll have to eat crow at least for a while until you take his (or her) place or are able to move on to another situation. Nevertheless, I will offer strategies to make your stressful situations less so and will offer physical and mental exercises for making such stressors less harmful to your health.

Introspection and Retrospection

At 40 you are at an age when you have already collected plenty of baggage. Some of it is good, and some of it—well, let's just put it this way: You'd just like to check it at the airport and hope it gets lost. It's been a long time since your world was new and your life was a blank slate where you would write all sorts of marvelous accomplishments.

At 40, instead of thoughts of the great deeds you *will* do, your mind can become a playground for demons, such as old failures, lost loves, bad bosses, awful jobs, and the big one—relationships with wives, children, and parents. If you're one of those guys who can simply put these gremlins out of your mind, then all the more power to you. But chances are that on occasion, almost anything can and will bother you.

Now, we all know that it's considered a guy thing to hide from your feelings. It's also considered unmanly to admit weakness, especially of the mental variety. What I suggest here is one coping method that you won't have to tell anyone else about. It's simply this: Think first. That's all. Go through any problem step by step and confront rationally the issues that are bothering you. Such analysis can serve a number of purposes, especially helping to identify exactly what is bothering you.

If you feel like talking about your struggle with someone, that's what friends are for. Impartial friends will do, lacking a local therapist or counselor. Or try writing about it. A note to a friend, a sibling, a parent, or your wife can sometimes be easier than a face-to-face or even phone conversation. In my case, writing an article about my mother's death helped me sort through what had been a stormy relationship. I described her last weeks, my role in them, and our conversations. It all helped me heal both from her death and from the problems we'd had between us over the years.

Yours will probably be a less public confession, but it could serve the same purpose. Get your feelings out in the open and explore what they mean to you, how you feel about them, and why they may hurt. Write first. Worry about sending it later. In fact, you may not want to send it at all. The therapy of just getting something down on paper (or on the computer, for that matter), something tangible, something outside your head, works wonders. In fact, women have known this for centuries, which is one reason (arguably) they are better adjusted than we are. Such personal exploration is one good way to stop old wounds from festering.

The best expert opinion I've found about dealing with life's many stresses is that trying to hide is futile. Thus your first four steps toward dealing with what seems to be an overwhelming problem are to

1. realize that other guys go through it too;
2. understand, however, that your troubles are still unique;
3. don't agonize over what you can't change; and

4. outwardly communicate about it with someone, even if that someone is yourself.

A Life Review Helps

Back in 1959, Erik Erikson, sometimes considered the father of the humanist school of psychology, stated that humanity's task "is to validate existence by seeing the past as meaningful." He argued that "the central dilemma for the aged is achieving integrity, a task that involves reconciliation to the personal past."

It is important to accept what life is all about, Erikson said, as well as to understand the people who are significant to us, without unrealistic wishes or regrets. For example, "It thus means a new and different love for one's parents, free of the wish that they should have been different and an acceptance of the fact that one's life is one's own responsibility."

Adding to Erikson's wisdom, Morton Lieberman and Sheldon Tobin, in *The Experience of Old Age: Stress, Coping, and Survival* (New York: Basic Books, 1983), advocate a life review as a method for finding inner peace, "a process involving psychic turmoil, confrontation of long-resolved conflicts, and effective extension of the self through time." Such a review, they state, produces "the integration of past conflicts, a high degree of life satisfaction, and serenity."

"The ability to engage in introspection on feelings during aging," Lieberman and Tobin argue, "may facilitate the formation of a strong self-concept in the present by providing a ready tool for integrating the remembered past and expected future." This means simply that looking back on our lives can give us a sense of connection between what we've been, what we are, and what we expect to become. In other words, reaching 40 may be a good time to reflect on past experiences in order to set a clear course for the future.

As it turns out, guys in their forties do plenty of introspection compared with those in their sixties or beyond, who have often done all the life review they need. In a sense, then, older individuals may well already have achieved peace on their journey. Another interesting finding is that the elderly create myths to dramatize their past. Lieberman and Tobin propose that "those who have resolved such a life review are more likely to experience equanimity, a sense of peace, and optimism about their future." Allowing you to create a comforting context to your life—even if it may be a "mythology"—may permit you to ultimately feel better about yourself.

A life review provides a uniqueness to your life by allowing you to define and defend your present self through a mythic review of your past. Have you ever noticed how seldom you reflect back on the bad times in your youth but instead remember all the great blasts you had in college?

(What about flunking introductory chemistry notwithstanding a planned career in medicine?)

Our cultural history is filled with special songs of past accomplishments. Is this bragging? Or is this a way of recognizing the important things men have done in their lives to become the people they are? The dialogue was often shared as something we gave each other—one man singing as friends listened. Now most of us live apart with walls between, physically and emotionally. Now friends aren't necessarily interested in such songs of our lives. That's not to say that we can't listen to our own diaries and gain from the experience, both from the compilation and the immersion in the process.

The hope is that once we accept our past as meaningful, we can feel less anxious about the future. Once we've honestly faced events that may have troubled us, these thorns can lose much of their deleterious power over us. Hopefully, content with what we may have done, we may perceive less pressure to do better or differently.

On occasion, however, some of these recollections can become too painful to bear. Yet often they are the ones that are most beneficial to resolve. This is called "facing your demons." Helping you do this is what analysts and counselors are for. In fact, processing your psychic confusion and pain is what they do for a living.

Reflecting on Your Feelings

There's an old saying that "women never know what they want; men never know how they feel." As men, we've long been taught that feelings are unmanly, and that to show emotion in a discussion or interaction is tantamount to being uncool, even unmasculine.

How we feel about things is important. A useful exercise in times of stress is to inventory your feelings. Let's say you're having a disagreement with your wife. Have you ever tried telling her simply and directly how you feel? I don't mean saying to her, "When you do this, *you* make me feel this way." That's not only untrue but irrelevant. Only *you* are responsible for your own emotions. Nobody else *makes* you feel anything. If she loves you, she will try to find a way to help keep you from feeling that way. But it isn't up to her to find a solution for your pain. It's up to you.

Here we are back to that struggle with feelings again.

A Time of Innocence

Ah, sweet youth wasn't so very long ago. Remember some of your youthful, childish behavior? Such as drinking until your stomach couldn't hold any more and your brain had regressed into the Stone Age? Or searching for that wild sexual adventure? Or experimenting with life-threatening exploits involving motorized vehicles, sporting equipment, controlled substances, or women?

Robert Bly would have us search for this hidden spirit within us by beating drums around a campfire. His discussions about such a search were never more poignant than in his dialogues with Bill Moyers. Bly discusses with Moyers how many of us have lost contact with our fathers. "Who were they?" Bly asks. Many of us never knew.

A lot of men have made similar pilgrimages in their lives. They find emotional benefit in reflecting on earlier innocent bondings in high school or college. Reexploring the sometimes bittersweet experiences of your turbulent earlier years can help you laugh at who you are today, not to mention the progression of history that has brought you to your present existence. It is not surprising that with time those experiences almost begin to feel as if they came from a different life, as if you were a different person then. And you know what? You probably were.

One realization you might come to is that not everything you did back then was stupid, although that may not be immediately apparent. Recall how important everything seemed back then—every political conflict, every test or paper, every social contact (especially the first ones), every disagreement with a roommate. All took on the gravity of the search for the Holy Grail. Only later could we allow ourselves to realize that the Grail was just a dusty beer mug, and that everything would turn out fine (if not great) nonetheless. We miss those days, even though we lacked the power and the gold that we may have today. Pity, we could have gotten into some real trouble if we did.

Political Solutions

As you get older, certain black beasts actually have their basis in public policy. A number of changes may even help you.

Demographers 20 or 30 years ago predicted that as the baby boomers approached and reached adulthood, they would swell the job market. With more workers available, these demographers theorized, actual work hours would decrease, and individual lives would become easier.

Needless to say, things didn't happen that way. Most people are working longer hours today than ever before, and the number of two-income households has exploded. In many instances, it has become easier, not harder, for an employer to exploit you. The way job stress affects you now is to make you worry all the more about whether you're going to have that raise in another six months—or even a job. Older workers face two disadvantages: Your experience means you command a greater salary, and your age dictates that you are more likely to need and use health care benefits. There are plenty of economic reasons why an employer may want to get rid of you. And they don't even include the built-in societal prejudice against older workers.

There is no easy solution here. In the short term, which is how most individuals confront their problems, we must be constantly vigilant against the worst-case possibilities to our careers. Planning is important. Working toward self-employment may be best for many, although it is unfortunately too often unrealistic.

The only reliable hope is to try to alter the characteristics of the workplace. Health care reform could go a long way toward ensuring the continued security of older workers. Employers, faced with increased health care costs from older workers, may be tempted to cut older workers loose. Should the burden of health care be lifted from employers, perhaps they will be far more likely to hold on to older and more experienced workers.

Depression Is an Illness!

Depression is an illness many of us must come to grips with in midlife. Depression can come as the product of genetic or emotional precipitating factors in our lives, perhaps expedited by one or more external events, but ending up with the potential to ruin jobs, families, and lives. In some cases, depression may actually have started earlier in our lives, masquerading through high school, college, and beyond as an inability to produce in school or at work or to perform successfully in one or another of life's relationships.

Depression is not a character weakness. It is a correctable, sometimes crippling condition that is probably inherited and certainly biochemically induced. It comes and goes elusively and, if uncontrolled, can kill. Medications such as older tricyclic antidepressants; newer, "cleaner" serotonin reuptake inhibitors such as Prozac, Paxil, and Zoloft; and lithium can restore energy levels and stabilize nasty mood swings. They are the keys that might break the cycle, the downward spiral of depression, and launch you back on the road to feeling good. It's more likely that such medications in conjunction with some sort of cognitive therapy will be necessary to bring you around to at least a level playing field from which to get better.

Recognizing and accepting depression as a bona fide disease is critical. Depression may not be a macho affliction, but without recognition and acceptance, either you'll never seek the help you need or you'll quit therapy or medication too early, risking your return to the abyss. So either be honest with yourself or find an impartial therapist who will act as your guide on your journey.

Some psychologists argue that healthy, positive memories of the past help to eliminate depression. One technique is to keep a journal. Libraries are filled with works by people who have chosen to publish and share their own life reviews. Another method is to join a men's group. Tell the group. Tell your wife or your lover what you have found out. Tell your bartender (that's a bartender's job, after all); tell your children; tell your best friend. They may squirm; they may fall asleep or try to leave the room. But if you're lucky, this process will be very familiar to all of them because as we slip and slide through one or another of life's rites of passage, almost everyone spends some time sharing his or her own brand of mortality, immortality, struggle, angst, or depression.

Sharing will ensure that you do not have to be alone. Those who share your honesty could help you appreciate how significant your struggle has been. Sure, there is a greater chance of exposing your own vulnerability. That's why you have to choose your sounding boards wisely. Remember that everyone has suffered in one way or another. Those closest to you can help you appreciate your own uniqueness and the value of your own life.

In return, you may have to listen to someone else's dirty laundry. There is no better way to ensure confidentiality than having shared someone else's innermost struggles. You often have to give to get, and it's worth it.

Stress Management

As I indicated earlier, stress is a throwback to prehistoric times when the body would secrete hormones, raise blood pressure, and in other ways prepare itself to deal with many dangers and challenges. In those days, these most basic biological responses were a simple matter of survival, because most emergencies were solved by killing or running away from something—the so-called fight or flight response.

We still have the same internal physical response, but in the modern world, the replacement stimuli tend to be situations that can't be dealt with simply by fighting or running away. In fact, many don't call for a physical reaction of any kind—including verbal. For this reason, stress is a complex mechanism with both physical and mental ramifications. More often than not, it must be dealt with mentally because dealing with the physical aspects of stress is, for the most part, considered to be dealing with the symptoms, not the cause.

Coping With Stress

The first line of attack taken by most experts is the assessment phase (called "psychological and emotional stress testing"). The degree of stress and, as much as possible, its causes, are defined. How do you really *feel*? With luck, your stress can be recognized, and you can start dealing with how stress affects you before it becomes too obvious—that is, before you suffer a stroke, a nervous breakdown, ulcers, or some other major physical or mental dysfunction.

Again, professional help is available for this critical phase in stress recognition and management. Here we are referring to psychiatrists, psychologists, or other mental health counselors.

The next level of approach is stress management itself. In any case, I strongly recommend that physical exercise be included in this phase for the simple reason that the absence of physical exercise is why stress builds up in the first place. If you lived in the Paleolithic Age, your stress would be caused by physical threats, and you would respond to them in a physical manner, thus dissipating the hormonal secretions and naturally allowing your body to return to its unstressed state. Also, although stress can be dealt with using drugs or other therapies, addressing symptoms, not causes, can lead to a Band-Aid approach.

In any long-term approach to stress management, relaxation is a key component. Various methods have been effective, ranging from transcendental meditation to biofeedback and psychological counseling. Yoga is effective not only for developing relaxation techniques but also for preparing the body before strenuous exercise. In this sense, yoga is used as a form of stretching.

Relaxation should be considered a complement to exercise, not a replacement, just as exercise must complement relaxation. Take your typical type A up-and-coming business wonk. Such an individual has never learned to relax easily. He thinks it's wimpy to relax. (Remember Michael Douglas's Gordon Gekko in the movie *Wall Street*? "Only wimps eat lunch.") Even his workouts are exercises in aggression and competition. He doesn't know how to achieve a relaxed state characterized by a decreased heart rate, blood pressure, oxygen consumption, muscle tension (EMG), electrodermal response, skin temperature, and nervous response. He probably wouldn't care even if he did recognize such a mellow state. That he was hyper was all the better to get the upper hand, to win, to screw the competition.

That exercise can facilitate relaxation is seemingly a paradox. But anyone who has experienced a night of passionate lovemaking or who has exercised heavily knows this is true. This is the body's own method for balancing itself. And the exercise (or the lovemaking) doesn't even need to be that intense. Even exercise of moderate intensity and duration relaxes muscle tension. What few men realize is that immediately following exercise, an optimal window for relaxation opens, whether it be in the sauna or hot tub or just simply meditating. In fact, it's a necessary component of healthy living, especially in avoiding postexercise arrhythmias and dysfunctional mood states. In other words, it's important to relax.

Getting in Touch to Calm Down

Type A behavior, with its screw-your-competitor, sell-your-own-mother mentality, may have been the preferred emotional behavior of the eighties, but as the millennium approaches, society is hopefully getting away from this self-destructive, self-indulgent, stress-creating behavior. Or at least some of us are trying. Can you change type A behavior? Studies have shown that people who participate in a regular exercise program can reduce their type A tendencies.

Many of the techniques employed with cardiac rehabilitation patients are applicable for specific stress management. One method is biofeedback-assisted relaxation training. Contrary to what too many people believe, you can control many of your so-called autonomic (or automatic) physiological responses to outside stimuli. In other words, you have the power to control not only voluntary behavior but also what has been considered to be involuntary behavior. Some of these involuntary behaviors include blood pressure, heartbeat, and galvanic skin response (GSR). Heightened levels of one or more of these can indicate stress. The theory is—and it appears to bear out—that if you can control these, you are in fact reducing the effects, such as heart disease, that a stressful life could be wreaking upon your body.

The problem is that many cardiac patients don't recognize when they're stressed out. For them, their stress baseline is much higher than that of others—that is, to them a high level of stress is normal. They may *think* relaxation, but their bodies are reacting otherwise.

Sound familiar?

Biofeedback employs modern learning techniques to teach the brain how to recognize and control even tiny amounts of change in heart rate, blood pressure, skin temperature, and GSR. The way biofeedback works is fairly simple. The body undergoes certain physiological changes in the body owing to stress. Two good examples are rising blood pressure and sweaty palms. Biofeedback trains you to recognize these responses as an indication of an increase in stress (or tension) and to use one of many relaxation techniques to reduce it.

Progressive Relaxation

The oldest method of stress reduction is called "progressive relaxation." Developed by Edmund Jacobson, it calls for alternately tensing, then relaxing certain muscle groups in the body. For example, you may begin with the feet, first tensing and relaxing the toes, then the foot itself, the ankle, the lower leg, and so forth until you reach the scalp. Once you have completed all the muscle groups, the overall effect can be total relaxation.

Another technique is "autogenic training," in which an individual brings back homeostasis to whatever system has gone awry. The key is self-suggestion and positive visualization. For example, blood flow can be increased to cold extremities by thinking "warm hands" or "warm feet." Headaches can be neutralized by consciously visualizing the draining of stress and tenseness from the head and body. Even high blood pressure and chronic pain have been reversed. Although this method takes sustained practice, those who practice it claim impressive results.

A third major method, called "breathing strategies," calls for achieving a relaxed state through slow abdominal breathing. This is the same technique used in Lamaze training for childbirth. Can millions of terrified couples be wrong?

A fourth method, "quieting reflex training," is similar to progressive relaxation, but rather than dealing with overall body relaxation, it employs a 6-second progressive relaxation process that is useful for mildly tension-provoking situations. As with progressive relaxation, one contracts various muscles throughout the body and then relaxes them. But because it's done relatively quickly, the process can be repeated hundreds of times a day for everything from mild to intensely stressful situations.

Finally, "cognitive restructuring" is a stress management procedure aimed at identifying and changing self-defeating and self-destructive thinking. This technique is a derivative of Albert Ellis's Rational Emotive Therapy. The goal is to transform thin-skinned and easily frustrated individuals into thick-skinned and emotionally stable people who can better fend off the stresses of daily life. Basically, it calls for ridding the mind of negative self-talk.

You can learn how to relax using one or another of these methods to deal more effectively with the tremendous number of emotional and physical stressors that constantly bombard you. Keep in mind that all these methods for relaxing have roots that are as old as civilization itself.

HOW TO CONTROL STRESS IN ONE EASY LESSON

Quickly relaxing while at your desk or at the wheel of your car in a traffic gridlock may help prevent elevations of those hormones that can attack your coronaries.

Incorporate relaxation into your stretching.

Learn techniques of relaxation as a means of coping with a stressful world.

Thomas Jefferson simply suggested counting to 10 or, if extremely agitated, to 100.

Coordinate Jefferson's with your own mantra breathing rhythm and you have pure Zen.

Ferraris, Gold Chains, and Your 23-Year-Old Secretary

Even though there are many techniques for dealing with stress, the bottom line is that you must deal with the stressors themselves, not just the symptoms. In all probability, your wife hasn't changed (at least no more than you have), and rush hour traffic will always be there, whether you're driving a Ferrari or a Yugo. Gold chains may or may not be flattering to you, but they hardly make you look younger, despite how much the chain costs.

Too often, those of us in midlife may engage in odd behavior because of fears or dissatisfactions about our lives, how we are aging, or what we may perceive lies ahead. Such angst is the subject of a plethora of cruel midlife jokes, as well as the cause of many divorces, and a boon to the U.S. government, thanks to import duties collected on impractical foreign cars.

Yet dealing with human behavior is never really simple. When the kids are graduated and gone, the time might seem perfect to end a relationship that has never been class A. Or a lot of families may have been broken up simply because a midlife man wanted to see how it felt again to sleep with a young woman, to preserve his perception of youth, to bathe, as it were, in the blood of virgins.

Whatever you do, make sure you know your motivations.

Buying fast cars, though it sounds silly, is probably one of the more harmless forms of midlife escapism. It's kind of like plastic surgery—if you can afford it and it makes you feel better about yourself, then what the hell?

On the other hand, why not deal with the source of the problem? If you feel good about yourself and accept your place in the world, then what does it matter what kind of car you drive or how old the woman is on your arm?

Remember what Polonius might have said: "To thine own self be true; which can certainly be cheaper and may also prevent a lot of litigation." (*Hamlet.* Act I, Scene 3. Really.)

Jim Bailey

From Texas to Tokyo

Just after college and looking for something to do with his life, Texas native Jim Bailey took off for Japan to teach English. Though it's not quite true that he never left, the experience forever changed his life. Now, nearly 30 years later, Jim considers himself more Japanese than American.

As a youngster moving from place to place—his dad could never quite find the right place to settle—Jim found himself attending one school after another, sometimes all in the same year. He still claims scars from the constant relocating, but by the time he started college, he found himself with a permanent home in Colorado. Tall, skinny, and not particularly athletic, he was considered by his friends to be a "brain" rather than a "jock." In fact, as a student at the Colorado College, he was on the school's GE College Bowl team.

Taking off for Tokyo after college put him yet again in a new location with few friends and lots of time. In a large city and without a car (which are enormously expensive in Japan), he naturally relied on his own two feet to get around. He also began attending a gym and began to work out. From then on, he parlayed his teaching into freelance writing, translating, and even modeling—quite a jump for the soft-spoken "brain."

Now a successful writer in two languages, Jim is married and has two children. Although Jim's wife, Yurika, and the kids live in the Seattle area (Yurika loves the American culture as much as Jim loves the Japanese), Jim divides his time between Tokyo and the West Coast, creating a thoroughly Pacific Rim family.

Because his writing life keeps him working long hours in front of a computer screen, Jim looks forward to his exercise time. His schedule includes a gym workout four days a week, 90 to 120 minutes at a time. He starts with 30 minutes on a stationary bike or treadmill and then follows that with a weight training program. He emphasizes the chest, shoulders, and triceps on one day, and the lats, biceps, and legs on another. With every session, he does abdominal exercises and lots of stretching. "Exercise," Jim says, "is a great stress reliever."

When in Tokyo, he still does not own a car and bikes or walks when he's not on the subway. And even though the Tokyo subway is a great system, it requires lots of bipedal activity to get between trains.

As for diet, Jim combines the best of West and East to maintain his 175 pounds on a 6'2" frame. Breakfast consists of half a grapefruit, a bowl of granola with yogurt, and a slice of bread with kiwi fruit slices on top. No butter, no jam. His lunches and dinner are more Japanese and include such staples as fish, tofu, steamed vegetables, and miso (bean paste) soup. Lately, he has deliberately cut down on his intake of sweets and rice.

He admits modestly that the trainers at his club say he has the body of man in his late twenties. He further notes that the asthma he's suffered from for past 20 years seems to have vanished, and he implies that it has done so as a result of his healthy lifestyle.

OK, Jim, so what is the secret of staying healthy and happy?

"Marriage," he says, noting the many studies that indicate that married men make out better in the health and happiness department than single guys. "Tolstoy observed that the only genuine happiness in this world comes from living for others. My own experience supports this: even while living the life of the carefree bachelor, I was constantly experiencing anxiety. With my wife and kids to take care of, I naturally have the worries any other male in same position undoubtedly has, but I derive enormous satisfaction out of what I'm doing on their behalf."

I couldn't have said it any better. But Jim, what about this long-distance relationship you have with them? You spend a lot of time literally a world apart.

Yes, he says, "I'm in Japan about eight months a year and am with my family in the States the remaining four. Fortunately, the fact that I'm busy helps me overcome loneliness. Knock on wood, my wife and I are still very much in love."

There you have it: Healthy living according to former Texan Jim Bailey. The magic formula is exercise, healthy diet, and lots of plain ol' lovin'.

Chapter 11

The Hazards
of Being 40
■ Overuse and Abuse

Middle age is the time when a man is always thinking that in a week or two he will feel as good as ever.

Don Marquis, U.S. humorist, journalist.
Quoted in E. Anthony, *O Rare Don Marquis*

Like any finely tooled machine, a 40-year-old body begins to break down. The trouble is that even efforts to improve this situation can result in problems.

This chapter deals with those hobgoblins that can afflict us as we exercise: overuse injuries, exercise asthma, runner's anemia, overtraining, the use and abuse of both prescription and nonprescription medications, and even exercise addiction—when what's good can become bad.

Injuries From Overuse

What is an overuse injury or problem, and why is it something to worry about as we get older? It usually is due to overloading and repetitive microtrauma (injury) to the musculoskeletal system—the result of *abuse, disuse, misuse,* and *overuse.* As sports medicine expert Jack Harvey, MD, so deftly explains: "Too much distance, too great intensity, or too much hill work." In other words, doing too much too soon or too often. A prime example is the would-be marathoner who does fine until he bumps up his mileage or speed. Then he risks the stress fracture that keeps him out of the Boston Marathon.

One common component of the list of overuse injuries includes painful stress fractures, especially involving the smaller bones of the feet or distal ends of the tibia or fibula. Type A behavior guys—you know, those who are compulsive—are prime targets for these overuse or self-abuse maladies.

Are you susceptible? Well, if you're popping all the Advil the local drugstore will sell you just to run through the pain, you'd better think hard about continuing at your current level of training.

Repetitive sports of any kind can wear out body parts. A good rule of

183

thumb to avoid such injuries is to remember the word *rotation*. In other words, rotate your sports *and* the ways you exercise.

For example, even top runners recommend against running every day. Your menisci, those two thin pads between your femur and tibia, may deteriorate. Also, if you're a former football player, buy your ticket early for your first arthroscopy—the procedure in which an orthopod (a bone specialist) looks into the knee joint and can repair such injuries as a meniscal buckle-handle tear.

Tendonitis is another frequent overuse injury of the lower extremities. The fascia lata, down the side of your thigh, is one of the most popular sites.

The severity of an overuse injury dictates the progression of pain. Does it begin at the start of exercise and then vanish, or does it continue and maybe worsen as the workout continues? Or does it occur only after exercising for a while? Or, worse yet, does it persist when you're not exercising?

Our compulsivity quotient often determines just how badly we end up injuring ourselves. Think prevention: Judiciously balance several different exercise disciplines—for example, stationary cycling, Nautilus, aerobics, running, and in-line skating. Another way to stay out of the infirmary of overuse injuries is to fold in some form of strength training, such as free weights, Nautilus, or good old push-ups, crunches, pull-ups, and other resistance exercises in your own backyard gym.

It should come as no surprise that overuse and stress injuries afflict those who fancy themselves top-level endurance athletes more than recreational athletes. Studies have indicated that endurance athletes experience three times more overuse injuries than do athletes in repetitive performance sports such as gymnastics.

AVOIDING OVERUSE

Think prevention: Build up exercise systematically. Take 10 minutes to warm up and don't forget to stretch both before and after your outing. You may want to secure advice from one of those well-muscled, happy guys who work in the weight room or even hire a personal trainer. Yes, these efforts take time away from your actual workout, but they are a much better investment than having to lay off for days, weeks, or even months because of injury.

Common Causes of Overuse Injuries

In general, overuse injuries are associated more with sports involving running and jumping. However, in spite of the obvious bang-thump qualities of such wonderful acts of gravitational defiance, overuse injures are more often due to intrinsic factors such as realignment or muscle imbalance in your feet. One common cause is pronation, a condition whereby the foot tends to roll over onto your instep, leading to a "toe out" walking or running style. (And we used to believe this was mostly hype to sell orthotics and more-expensive running shoes.)

Excessive pronation can progress to increased internal rotation of the entire leg, putting painful torque on the Achilles tendon or the patellofemoral ligament (the one that attaches your kneecap to your upper leg).

There are many other sources of such injury. The career of the great St. Louis Cardinal pitcher Dizzy Dean, for example, was ended by a foot injury that altered his motion just enough to ruin his pitching arm. In short, performing a sport or exercise wrong can be a prime cause of overuse injury. This is where a good coach or trainer comes in.

But it's not the only way. Overuse injury can be just that—an overdoing of a potentially injurious motion or workload on a part of your body. Repeatedly pounding the knee with hard-pavement running, for example, even if you're doing it just right, can hurt you eventually.

RUNNER'S HIGH

Runner's high is a condition that often affects better-conditioned athletes. It typically hits after several months of training, 30 to 40 minutes into a regular aerobic workout. Some runners live for it, and it does you absolutely no harm. The state may be described as one of mastery, patience, openness and capacity for change, distraction, altered consciousness, and realization (eureka!) of one's potential.

Studies have attributed runner's high to the active opiate-like peptides in the brain also known as beta-endorphins and meta-encephalins. These hormones, which increase with exercise, may favorably affect up to three out of four fit runners. Beta-encephalins, similar peptides, are secreted by the pituitary, the so-called master gland, at the base of the brain.

So what do these endorphins do? When similar substances are injected, they produce analgesia, a state of numbness, and a certain freedom from pain. They also can produce a cataleptic state with a reduction in response to external stimuli.

Other researchers attribute runner's high to neurotransmitters such as epinephrine and serotonin. But no matter what the cause, the effect is often stunning: Some runners even report mystical experiences in which colors intensify, clouds dance, worries disappear, and grand ideas happen. It's almost too bad that runner's high can't be bottled and sold over the counter at your local pharmacy.

Exercise Addiction

Although exercise is good, overdoing it can be bad. In most cases, the result of too much exercise is a physiological problem, but in some, it becomes psychological. This is what we call exercise addiction. Put simply, exercise addiction occurs when an athlete cannot get his exercise "fix" and begins to experience exercise withdrawal. The result, as in any addiction, is personal havoc.

How do you know if you're an exercise addict? Honestly answer the questions in the following test:

1. Is the rest of my life secondary to my sport (or exercise)?

| | Yes | No | Maybe |

2. Am I choosing my sport (or exercise) over my family or other close personal relationships?

| | Yes | No | Maybe |

3. Am I compelled to practice my sport (or exercise) even when I am injured or in pain?

| | Yes | No | Maybe |

4. If I cannot practice my sport (or exercise) do I always become irritable or antisocial?

| | Yes | No | Maybe |

5. Does my sport (or exercise) distract me from my work or from making a living?

| | Yes | No | Maybe |

If you answered "yes" or "maybe" to just one of these questions, you need to reexamine closely your relationship with your exercise regimen. This is when you may want to visit your health care clinic and have a discussion with your physician or nurse practitioner. Or you may want to consult with a mental health specialist such as a psychiatrist or psychologist. After all, an addiction, no matter how good its original purpose, if brought to these extremes is still an addiction.

As with alcoholism, the effects of exercise addiction often show up last in the workplace. In fact, your work may be a great reinforcer for an exercise addiction. Colleagues may admire you for your commitment to running, skiing, or biking. On the other hand, wives, children, or lovers will be the first to notice that something isn't quite right.

Dr. Rob Johnson, a running enthusiast and sports medicine expert at the Hennepin County Department of Family Practice and Sportsmedicine Program in Minneapolis, prefers the term "exercise dependence" over "exercise addiction." He qualifies "dependence" as physiological and "addiction" as psychological. An addicted (or dependent) athlete who stops exercising for whatever reason reports anxiety, irritability, restlessness, apathy, sluggishness, weight gain or loss, decreased appetite, sleep problems, headaches, stomachaches, cramps, guilt, tension, and bloating. (It is hard to get much more physiological than that.) A short tour of any city hospital will offer similar withdrawal symptoms in drug addicts and alcoholics. Given the choice between withdrawal and pain, it is no wonder that some athletes keep churning out the miles despite the threat of further injury or the destruction of their personal lives.

Johnson defines an exercise-dependent person as someone who
1. maintains a rigid exercise pattern,
2. places exercise above other activities,
3. must exercise more to achieve the same high,
4. experiences severe withdrawal symptoms if he stops, and
5. returns quickly to compulsive exercising after a break.

Overtraining

We've all heard of this, but what the hell is it? This difficult phenomenon often surfaces as a plateau in performance. Such "staleness" is endemic to the endurance sports of cycling, distance running, rowing, cross-country skiing, and swimming. The symptoms of "going flat" from overtraining can include
1. slowed performance,
2. muscle pain (myopathy),
3. elevated blood pressure and morning pulse,
4. sleep problems ranging from restlessness and inability to sleep to chronic fatigue or tiredness,
5. appetite problems ranging from lack of appetite to bingeing and bulimia,
6. elevation of the muscle enzyme creatine phosphokinase (CPK) due to muscle injury or destruction, and
7. dysphoria such as anxiety or depression.

What is the antidote? The hardest prescription an athlete can hear is "rest," even if only temporarily. This is when the athlete's "bereavement skills" must surface—coping techniques which he, unfortunately, might finally have to learn to develop.

Runner's Anemia

If you're a runner, anemia is something you probably want to watch carefully for one big reason: Any kind of iron deficiency anemia means an aggressive search for signs of blood loss from the gastrointestinal tract. As I've mentioned in previous chapters, blood in the bowel can indicate any number of unpleasant problems, including colitis, polyps, fissures, hemorrhoids, tears, and the Big One, colon cancer.

One of the problems with overexercising is that you can develop a condition that can masquerade as something worse than it really is. Here's the litany.

Many runners will tell you (often sheepishly) about some very unpleasant side effects that occur usually during times of rapid increase in training or races. These include "runner's trots," abdominal cramping, bloating, frequent BMs, and watery stools. In fact, there is something like an 80 percent decrease in blood flow to the gut while running, especially among those of us who are less well trained. In athletes and duffers alike, running hard is enough to produce ischemia (temporary, localized anemia) of the bowel, which can produce bleeding. Many athletes compound this condition by abusing aspirin or other nonsteroidal anti-inflammatories with very much the same effect—microbleeds, gastritis, and ultimately an iron deficiency anemia.

When blood started showing up in the urine of a group of Norwegian cadets, doctors were at first puzzled. Eventually the cause was determined to be hemolysis (destruction of red blood corpuscles) from repeated marching on hard pavement. Thus, the condition came to be called March Hematuria. Other studies have shown hematuria (blood in the urine) among distance runners due to trauma to the posterior bladder and iron deficiency anemia due to a loss of red cells from ischemic kidneys. Another problem, especially in young, highly exertional athletes, is a hidden blood loss from the bowels due to intestinal ischemia (stress gastritis).

When you're over 40, make sure you check your blood count yearly—especially if you exercise. Generally, there are simple tests to determine whether you suffer from anemia and, if so, what that anemia is. In any event, if exercise does cause bleeding, get thee to a medical care specialist pronto and find out what's going on.

Exercise Asthma

Exercise-induced asthma (EIA) is a real clinical entity, according to Dallas sports medicine expert Dr. Jim Stray-Gundersen. When confronted with cold, dry air, most athletes will develop bronchoconstriction (wheezing on expiration), labored breathing (dyspnea), and at least some coughing. EIA is an increase in airway resistance, especially in the smaller muscular breathing tubes, that typically comes on 5 to 10 minutes after exercising. It can also can occur during maximal exertion.

What causes it? The experts have shown that EIA results from increased respiratory heat exchange or water loss from the lining of the airways. Hyperventilating because of physical or psychological factors then triggers fragile mast cells to burst and release their trigger substance—histamine. This constricts the smooth, muscle-lined airways and produces bronchospasm. It can be made worse if you're predisposed from, let's say, a preceding upper respiratory infection or irritation from ambient pollutants or smoking.

Now for the good news.

Fit asthmatics actually bronchodilate better than unfit asthmatics. This is true for both EIA and regular asthma. Certainly, a sport such as swimming, in which the athlete breathes moist, warm air, should be easier on a touchy pulmonary system.

Athletes who suffer from EIA will often wear a face mask, particularly during the refractory, or warm-up, phase of training. Alternatively, they will choose to warm up inside before venturing into arctic air. A sufficient warm-up during the refractory period stabilizes the mast cells for at least an hour. Consequently, they won't release histamine as soon as you hit the cold air. One Olympic silver medalist says that coping with EIA is mostly just a matter of common sense and staying in tune with your body.

Drug Reactions and Exercise

Although it's always wise to think carefully about what prescription and nonprescription drugs may do to your body, it's even more important as you get up in years. Many common over-the-counter (OTC) and prescription remedies have some pretty heavy-duty side effects.

One option before swallowing one or another panacea is to consult a book such as *The Essential Guide to Prescription Drugs* by James W. Long, MD. Or try to find a physician who is willing to serve as a telephone resource. Your pharmacist should be more than happy to provide information on the medications your doctor has prescribed.

Let's run through some of the more common medications.

We'll start with antidepressants. One class, tricyclics such as imipramine, may resurrect us from the pits of depression, but at a price. The downside can be low blood pressure and either rapid heart rate (tachycardia) or irregular rhythm (arrhythmia). Other side effects from antidepressants in this class include sleepiness, constipation, urinary retention, and blurred vision.

The good news is that there is a group of antidepressants in the fluoxetine class (Prozac, Zoloft, Paxil, and others), which are chemically unrelated to the other antidepressants and lack many of their bothersome side effects. Aside from weight loss, headaches, or stomach distress if taken on an empty stomach, these medications are as side effect free as any strong drug can be.

Another group of antidepressants, the MAO inhibitors, are usually reserved as a last resort. There is a significant chance this drug will react with foods containing tyramine, such as aged cheese, beer, wine, or chocolates, which can precipitate a hypertensive crisis.

Lithium, either alone or with one of the newer "clean" antidepressants such as Prozac or Zoloft, can prevent violent mood swings symptomatic of the bipolar illness manic-depression. It is imperative for anyone taking lithium to have his level checked frequently until stable and then periodically thereafter (every three to six months). Those on lithium should be prepared to gain weight either from suppression of thyroid function or a decreased metabolic rate (BMR). Kidney function can also become compromised and should be evaluated periodically.

Xanax, one of the benzodiazepams like Valium or Librium, not only has anxiolytic (anxiety-lessening) capacity but also has quick-acting antidepressant qualities. Therefore, Xanax can mollify agitated depression while a tricyclic antidepressant is kicking in. It is not unusual for an antidepressant to take two or three weeks before it starts working. The negative side of Xanax is that it can be habit-forming. A physician will prescribe it only for a limited period. Individuals unfortunate enough to have panic attacks, however, may have to take this medication indefinitely.

The anti-inflammatories such as aspirin or ibuprofen work quite well for most people. Americans gulp down a hundred million aspirin daily. Aspirin products that are prevalent in such old standbys as Anacin or Alka-Seltzer are analgesic, anti-inflammatory, and antipyretic (fever suppressants). Acetaminophen (such as Tylenol) is not an anti-inflammatory, but it does just fine for pain or fever.

Don't forget that indiscriminately popping nonsteroidal anti-inflammatory drugs (NSAIDs) such as Motrin and Naprosyn can, like aspirin, produce microbleeds in the stomach. Aspirin inhibits platelet adherence or "stickiness" in the blood. Although taking one baby aspirin a day can be an excellent prophylactic way to prevent clotting and strokes, one should avoid aspirin products immediately after soft-tissue injuries when there is the danger of painful bleeding into those tissues, thus producing a hematoma.

The treatment of hypertension can include the use of the beta-blocker propranalol (Inderal). This is also a superb medication for angina, heart rhythm problems, migraines, anxiety, or stage fright. However, it can slow the heart or precipitate asthma. It shouldn't be used by anyone who has heart failure or diabetes. Some side effects include fatigue, depression, and bizarre dreams.

The cardiac vasodilators and calcium channel blockers effectively dilate the coronaries and decrease afterload, or the pressure against which the heart must pump. Nitrates not uncommonly produce pesky headaches or postural hypotension (drops in blood pressure). Some of the calcium channel blockers can cause constipation, and any antihypertensive can produce hypotension.

If you're on certain water pills for heart failure, it is important to replenish your supply of potassium. If your kidneys are functioning normally, you can consume as much potassium as available. But if you are losing a great deal of potassium or you are on diuretics, make sure you consume foods high in potassium, such as bananas, freshly squeezed orange juice, and potassium-rich veggies. Hypokalemia (low potassium) from excessive use of diuretics can lead to decreased muscle strength, work performance, and blood volume, as well as muscle cramps, orthostatic hypotension, and cardiac rhythm disturbance.

You should also know that tetracycline or sulfa-containing antibiotics like Bactrim can produce hypersensitivity to the sun. The result can be a serious sunburn on your next outing to the beach.

Although this is only a partial list of medicines men over 40 take, there are plenty of other resources. Ask your physician, nurse practitioner, or pharmacist. Invest in one of the many books on common medications. Medical reference CDs make wonderful reference tools for your computer. Even the Internet offers many resources.

Check and double check. The bottom line is to be responsible for your own health and medications. Isn't that why you're reading this book?

Sudden Death—Reprise

We hear from time to time about someone who is theoretically in perfect health but drops dead while exercising. Though I covered the notions of heart attack and other sudden knockout punches in chapter 1, this subject bears another look in the context of how much—if at all—fear of death should inhibit you from undertaking an exercise program.

To review: For those of us who are still under 35, the most likely cause of sudden death while exercising is from a congenital abnormality of the heart. This includes anomalous coronary vasculature where, for instance, the right coronary artery supplies the large left ventricle. Other possibilities include Marfan's syndrome, aortic stenosis, and atrial or ventricular septal defects. Many of these conditions can be detected historically or with a physical exam.

Past age 35, the predominant danger is arteriosclerotic coronary vascular disease (ASCVD). This could mean anyone with a strong family history of heart disease (as evidenced by heart attacks or strokes), hypertension, or diabetes, or anyone who has a history of smoking. Look for hyperlipidemia (high triglyceride and cholesterol) levels. Here's when you need to get a stress test.

It is likely that much of the physical deterioration in functional capacity of the elderly is due to culturally induced inactivity. In other words, if you don't use it, you will lose it.

When we think of dropping dead while exercising, the name of Jim Fixx comes quickly to mind. This pioneer of the running revolution of the 1970s, as we all know, dropped dead while on a pleasant run on a country road. The press, ever vigilant for an easy chance to tarnish the image of a well-respected athlete, had a field day.

But there's more to the story. Formerly a heavy smoker, Fixx earlier had warning symptoms of heart problems. He had complained of radiating chest, neck, arm, and cheek pain while exercising, while shaving in the morning, and while driving the car (so-called executive angina). There were hereditary factors as well. He apparently failed to heed suggestions by Ken Cooper on a visit to the author's aerobic institute with the late George Sheehan. George did listen to Cooper. Though he had prostate cancer, he managed to live successfully for over a decade. Jim didn't and ended up dropping dead on his last run. On autopsy, he had three-vessel disease and a severely damaged left ventricle—a condition easily found within minutes by just running on a treadmill.

It's easy to ask: Why were you so stubborn, Jim, not to get tested properly? Not to acknowledge these symptoms? We'll never know. But in spite of his challenged cardiovascular system, his last years were active and enjoyable. Perhaps the man simply didn't want to live his life as a heart cripple. Perhaps he knew he was at a disadvantage anyway, so why not do what he liked? There's certainly the possibility that he might have died even earlier had he not launched into his later-life exercise regimen. It was, after all, his choice.

It's Your Choice

We're all faced in a greater or lesser way with the same choice as Jim Fixx. And the statistics are a bit confusing. On the one hand, vigorous exercise does actually increase your chance of dying suddenly, usually from a fatal arrhythmia. This is how college basketball player Hank Gathers died, but there were certain complicating issues such as an arrhythmia responsive to the beta-blocker Inderal. The opposite side of the coin is that regular exercise over time does, in fact, decrease your chances of dying suddenly and prematurely and definitely improves the quality of your life.

So here's the skinny: If you are over 35, get a baseline cardiogram. Evaluate a fasting blood specimen for cholesterol and triglycerides. Throw in a urine sample. You'd be pissing it away anyway, and it's a quick way to find protein, sugar, or blood.

To repeat what I said in the first part of this book, if you think you have any of the risk factors, bite the bullet and get a supervised maximal stress test. This type of study can detect correctable coronary artery disease. If there is any question about the results, depending on the cardiologist's suspicions, other noninvasive tests such the thallium scan and the echo stress test can be performed before an angiogram is considered necessary.

The goal of exercising must not be simply to add years to our lives, but life to our years. We live in a society that has made a science of culturally induced inactivity; Americans are great watchers but lousy doers. And, yes, "doing" offers some risk. But whether that risk comes from overuse, overtraining, exercise addiction, sportsman's anemia, exercise-induced asthma, or "instant death," the following admonition holds true: Simply know where the line is and avoid crossing it.

The overwhelming evidence is that your life can be better if you opt for a life of action.

Bob Fischbeck

Salesman

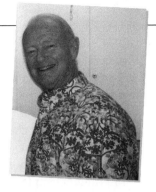

Bob Fischbeck neither looks nor acts like a guy in his seventies. He's fit, tanned, muscular, and a bundle of energy. Pretty good for a guy who, if genetic history were the determining factor, ought to be dead.

Bob's been in the steel business all his life. And for most of his career, he lived the by-the-book salesman's life: lots of eating on the road, plenty of cocktails, the usual push, push, push for the next sale. But he was always cognizant of one thing: None of his male relatives lived very long, usually because of the effects of high blood pressure. His father, in fact, died from a stroke at the age of 62.

In 1984, at the age of 60, Bob finally realized that he had to do something about his growing gut and elevating blood pressure. He decided to make the toughest sale of his life: He had to sell himself on getting healthy. He knew he had to shape up or forget it.

He chose to shape up. He quit drinking, cut down on the steak dinners on the road, and began going to the gym.

It wasn't all that easy at first. His initial visits to the gym were very tentative. He remembers going to a Gold's Gym in Southern California, walking in, and after seeing all the beefy guys doing weights, walking out again. But he realized he couldn't be intimidated. He had to start sometime, and that time was now. So he turned around and went back. As he walked in the door, one of the guys in the gym asked if he could help Bob out. The master salesman who hardly admits to any frailty confessed that he didn't know what he was doing. The guy said, "Come on. I'll show you." That was Bob's first experience with a personal trainer.

"A lot of guys who are first starting out worry about what the people in the gym will think about them," Bob says. "The answer is: They're respected. The guys in the gym realize that we all have to start out somewhere."

Bob says that having a personal trainer early on in his weight training gave him the confidence not to be intimidated. And over the years, he has learned that the two keys to continued success are having the right attitude and being consistent. You can't stop and start, stop and start. To stay fit, you have to keep at it.

Today Bob still works out in the gym 5 days a week for 2 hours, usually between 5:00 and 7:00 P.M. That includes bike riding or the treadmill, and a session with free weights. When he's on the road selling, he maintains this regimen, finding he can access gyms wherever he is for $5 or $10 a visit—sometimes for no charge if there's a reciprocal agreement with his own gym.

Diet is also important to Bob's theory of beating the genetic odds. For breakfast he usually has shredded wheat and fresh fruit or juice. When on the road, he shuns fast food. As for healthy dinners, he credits his wife, Kathy. "She's a great cook, you know," he says, citing curried chicken rice as just one of her specialties. "You don't lose your gut by doing sit-ups. It's what you put in your mouth," he says.

After teetotaling for a while, Bob is back to an evening cocktail and sometimes wine with dinner. His father-in-law was a hell of a martini maker, and Bob follows in this tradition. But he has given up his periodic cigar. And in deference to those genes and modern medicine, he takes blood pressure medicine daily.

At 73, Bob Fischbeck is as healthy and happy as he's ever been. This master salesman is just one guy who every day is beating the odds.

Chapter 12

Spirituality
■ **Try It, You'll Like It**

The soul, like the body, lives by what it feeds on.

Josiah Gilbert Holland

At 40, we're all entering a very fragile time in our lives. It only takes a quick peek in the mirror any morning to see more gray hair—or just less hair. Those pecs aren't as well-defined as they were when we were in college a quarter of a century ago—in fact, they're probably downright saggy.

Any spirituality we may have possessed in that younger life may not be as relevant as it was then. The spirituality that may have worked for us while our parents were still alive and while we were part of their family unit may no longer suffice. Just witnessing the decline in our parents can produce increasing fears about our own mortality. With parents increasingly out of the picture due to death, senility, or geographic separation, we may no longer feel the same pressure to continue their religious beliefs, especially in this land of the free and the brave.

That may take many routes. There is, for example, a significant renaissance within the "yuppie" Jewish community to locate its own spiritual roots. Black and Native American ethnicity as well as Hasidic, Muslim, and Christian fundamentalism speak to up-and-coming generations in search of their souls. It is increasingly up to each of us to locate a spirituality that will work for us and our growing families. Such a search can frequently begin on the track, in the swimming pool, in the gym, on the slopes, or on the road over humming spoked wheels, often under the rubric of finding, relocating, or just maintaining our health.

In *Seasons of a Man's Life,* the late psychologist Daniel Levinson emphasizes that many men "neurose" about the direction of their lives during their twenties and thirties. He notes how men may struggle for meaning in what they are doing at this stage rather than later, in their forties and fifties—when, he says, it counts more. Yet a search for meaning later in life is every bit as meaningful as all that time and effort we devoted to the same task in high school or college. Now there can be a renewed vigor, a passion modulated, as it were, by some glimpse many of us may have had of our fragility, our mortality.

Studies at Harvard University indicated that participating on the Crimson football team had far less to do with preventing later morbidity and mortality than continued exercise—that is, prodding our aging bodies into action in our later decades. There is likewise a similar need, I suspect, to probe a spiritual center inside each of us also to help us deal with our angst that we will drop dead in bed, while running, making vigorous love, or, as in the case of one extremely healthy friend and patient of mine in his mid-thirties, while sitting on the biffy on a friend's sailboat on Lake Superior.

I am continually reminded of the title of Dr. Harold S. Kushner's book, which emphasizes that it is not *why* but *When Bad Things Happen to Good People*. There is often no explanation why a phenomenon such as sudden death arbitrarily takes one perfectly fine person but leaves behind some really rotten son of a bitch. My father often said, "Life isn't fair."

Spirituality and Exercise

One simple way to search for inner peace in this life (the only one we've got, at least according to my religion) may be something as simple as a 45-minute run, a winter ski tour, a vigorous game of racquetball, or an hour's rollerblade along a state trail that was once an old paved railroad bed. Exercise can be a mantra, an escape, a way to process unsettling thoughts, an opportunity for exploring ideas, or a method to resolve problems with loved ones, friends, or fellow workers. Unfortunately, such escape via a cleansing internal dialogue may allow some of the same struggles to continue to live inside the brain or escape. Is such preoccupation with exercise all too Western or, I fear, not altogether spiritual? Techniques involving repetitive physical movements may still be the best escape, the best catharsis, the vehicle that can take you furthest from your angst and help to release you from those "civilized" chains you wear. It can be your Western mantra.

There must be some reason why so many men, as they reach their forties, feel compelled to run their first marathon, become a first-time triathlete, leap out of perfectly good planes over verdant rural countryside, or bungee jump from tall bridges. It is during this sometimes painful period that men may find themselves chanting such mantras as "no pain, no gain" and "use it or lose it." They suddenly discover that they are in search of "the word" or "the ideal," or simply the answer to the question "Why the heck am I doing what I'm doing every day?"

Many of us think that because we decided to enter a lofty profession such as medicine, law, or teaching, we have attained the priesthood. Not so. There are a battalion of naysayers out to dethrone us. Whatever we do is just a job. We are who we are, not what we do.

Yes, life is madness, but now it carries a different theme than the one that motivated us during the sixties and seventies. There is a new modus operandi: It is better to scale peaks, accomplish new personal bests, and push for success (whatever that means) than to keep sexual scores, drink to oblivion, go for days without sleep, or sample every new hallucinogen on the market. Hey, you haven't forgotten about AIDS, have you?

Discovery

It wasn't until I began a committed relationship with Suzy, the woman who would become my wife, that I truly first began to get inside my own sensuality and understand the spirituality and beauty of my relationship with just one life partner. Yet having children was what truly first taught me how to love. I had to learn—and it wasn't entirely easy—how to balance exercise and competition with an understandably demanding relationship with a wife and three young girls. My exercising and competitive frenzy would often serve as an escape from that very intimacy. (Just ask my wife.) The consequence of my own sometimes self-abusive habits would affect my mood until I could be nearly impossible to live with. (Just ask my kids.) Consequently, I had to learn how to modify this wish to escape physically and emotionally from my pain so as not to make the stress worse on me or my family.

The necessity for discovering or rediscovering the soul in our primary relationships is of tantamount importance. In *Care of the Soul,* Thomas Moore emphasizes just how necessary it is to continue a search for the spirit in our relationships and also how out of control this search can become.

For many unfortunate reasons, one friend and his wife, a decade into a successful marriage that had produced two beautiful children, discovered that they had very much lost perspective on the soul of their relationship. Meeting another woman, with whom this friend soon came to spend many weekends cycling, began as an innocent opportunity to teach and share his sport with her and her son. It wasn't long before this liaison made him aware of how much he felt he was missing in his own relationship, making him crave the same kind of soul in his own life as he had discovered illicitly on weekends with his new friend.

He was sharing with another woman not only his passion for cycling but also the spirituality he felt in his sport. She was willing to join him on his search while his own wife understandably was preoccupied with a new career and their children. Here was his chance to share an escape from the stressors of a demanding legal career.

As Moore has suggested, the friend fortunately realized just how much he wanted passion back in his primary relationship. This other woman was a dangerous replacement for what he later realized was missing in his own world. He soon resolved to try to find spiritual peace at home.

Moving On

The forties can be a time to try competition as a legitimate challenge separate from work. In the work environment, a snake pit for many, you may have conquered all that you felt you ever could or vanquished everyone you always wanted. Perhaps you have discovered you have nowhere else to go in your profession. It can be a startling realization that no matter how valuable you may have thought your chosen career goal was, it's just a job.

Although competition may provide a vital stimulus lacking in your life, it can offer a downside. Remember, competition is no substitute for spirituality. If competition becomes its own seductive religion, it can supplant other important things in life, including more valid routes to spirituality. Instead, what you may end up doing by taking up competition becomes understandably overplanned or, by necessity, overrehearsed.

The mind-set required of those who shove feet into starting blocks is often called an "iceberg personality." Translation: Any connection to anything other than positive, unwavering, and undistracted strength within your spirit is verboten. Only one person can come in first. Sure, other poor slobs can take second or third, but the accolades will never go to them.

The demands of building a career while maintaining some semblance of success as an involved father eliminate competition for many, especially men who have young children or working wives. Yet competition can be as addictive as any controlled substance. Nonetheless, many men lust for spirituality in the process of competition, only to realize that the end result does not afford much opportunity to smell the flowers or peer within themselves to explore issues of "Why?"

A successfully focused adherent of yoga can learn ways to separate from physical pain by creating a deep trancelike state. High-level athletes have admitted they would willingly opt for certain death in 10 years just to win an Olympic medal. Perhaps such intensity (or addiction) explains why top-level athletes have chosen to train unmercifully or to take steroids, speed, or dope despite the dangers.

Smelling the flowers is every bit as sensual and spiritual an experience. Running or hiking over a full shock of wet earth, by a swamp, near blossoming lilies, or through a forest with every sort of spring flower bursting within touch can impart an awareness that there is a larger force out there that has started the whole parade rolling.

A search for spirituality can end up being very different for all of us. One father in his sixties explains that he finds his nirvana through music and by being with his family. "One thing I have done," he says, "was to join a book group at our church. I don't go to church very often. I read, but I wouldn't necessarily read these kind of books if it weren't for being in this group." This is the same father and husband who has become what *Zen and the Art of Motorcycle Maintenance* is all about: Over the past two decades, he has been building and racing cars and motorcycles. Two of his three daughters are accomplished professional jazz singers, and he spends plenty of time going to hear them sing at one venue or another.

THE RUNNING RABBI

A rather erudite rabbi I know and admire surprised me after I told him that I had very little interest in group worship.

"I wouldn't want to go to temple either," he said with complete seriousness, "if I weren't a rabbi." This same rabbi, I might add, although a mere wisp of a man, runs around our lakes religiously all seasons of the year.

This story alludes to some of my own struggle with traditional Judaism and organized religion. Accomplishing my Bar Mitzvah was no small challenge. The rabbi kept on threatening to kick me out if I didn't behave. But my acting out had to do with the fact that I could not relate to either this rabbi or a liturgy I could not understand. Yet the Judaism of my Bar Mitzvah did unite my extended (tribal) family, if only for a day or two, and may have helped me better understand my culture. Put simply, it was a rite of passage and the affirmation of becoming an adult in my own family system (tribe).

Universality

A love of sport crosses cultural and ethnic lines. Equally fascinating are a Brit like Harold Abrahams (biographed in the film *Chariots of Fire*), winner of the 100-meter dash in the 1924 Paris Olympics, and Irving Jaffee, winner of two Olympic gold medals at the 1932 Lake Placid Olympics in the 5,000- and 10,000-meter speed skating competitions. Abrahams, like myself, came from comfortable means; Jaffee's father had operated a pushcart. However, both athletes labored successfully to bring different gifts to their chosen sport despite anti-Semitism and athletic xenophobia from fellow athletes. Jaffee, for instance, initially never considered ice-skating because he saw it as a Nordic sport, "one definitely not for Jews." However, both found their inner answer and self-definition—their spirituality and preeminence—through competition in running and ice-skating in a world that thought, "right God, wrong church" about anyone who did not happen to be Christian.

Deepak Chopra recommends not only daily meditation for greater inner peace, but also a cleansing walk in the woods (or some place quiet and natural) away from your life stressors. These days I prefer to escape the driving pace of my life in the woods either on my skis, hiking with my ski poles, or, if I'm really energetic, running up and down a trail in my favorite woods.

I like the image that Bruce Dern, himself a marathoner, espouses as he dramatizes preparing for a race from the mountains to the sea so that he can soar up the hills like an eagle and float back down like a feather. Again, I think we are looking at a quest for inner peace that sometimes can be accomplished by athletically challenging our lungs or hearts. Who knows how much of our pleasure is derived from endorphins and how much from plain distraction from all the turmoil of life? While still at Dartmouth, my roommate (now New York surgeon) Dr. "Kip" Minaert and I fantasized that we would become Olympic flat-water canoe champions. What we gained from our daily training trips canoeing up and down the Connecticut River provided necessary quiet from the storm of our pre-med studies.

We must find ways within ourselves, and perhaps by whatever healthy escape technique we can muster, to separate ourselves from the stress of day-to-day existence. I personally see little difference from Eastern-style meditation and consistently exercising. Perhaps your meditation can be walking three times a week, creating your own special mantra by repetitively peddling a bike, or just the slow, deep breathing of fresh air while canoeing or kayaking.

ON BEING ALONE

I have felt some of my life's most cleansing moments floating out as far as I can go in a nearby lake and feeling the cold springs shoot up against my body. Or counting over and over the number of steps I have taken climbing a hill or speed skating over a country road or path. All of this helps distract me from what I want to put aside for the hour I have consciously chosen to feel my body, sense the water, and touch the earth.

At this point in my life, I have little interest in organized worship. A principal reason for my philosophy is that I have little use for religions that permit the slaughter of innocents in the name of some special notion of God. I have chosen to seek the pleasure of achieving fitness, which has allowed me to sail breathlessly through forests or to run along quiet country roads. Entering the private world of deer and other animals and gathering morels or berries as I hike are just fringe benefits of such luxurious escapism into the quiet world of exercise and the outdoors.

There's no limit to what can occupy the mind while the body is in the act of exercising repetitively and comfortably. The runner's high is an example of an exercise-induced pleasure zone for those who are willing to devote enough time to the sport—at least 6 months, 30 to 40 minutes a day. Some say such a high is the stuff of an altered mind, not too dissimilar from what others achieve with meditation or prayer.

So, it's no surprise that there may be a lot in common among traditional communal worship, transcendental meditation, and escaping into the woods for a long, unfettered hike or ski. Many insist that they have found God while hanging upside down scaling a mountain. Others may find Allah at the top of their favorite downhill run or as they soar down this same trail emotionally unencumbered, dealing with such a complex and challenging activity as simple survival.

Men are often as negligent about meditating as they are with stretching before, and especially after, exercise. There is every reason to believe that short periods of meditation (or some of the pleasurable escape thoughts learned on the trail or on a bike) can help impart relaxation skills to erase your stressors as they arise throughout the day. One communications expert has suggested how valuable a quick cleansing breath can be between clients. There is much to be gained by using Eastern skills in our daily Western lives. The best athletes have been doing this for some time.

A simple Western alternative is to develop your own mantra while running, swimming, rollerblading, or hitting the tennis ball to help make whatever form of exercise you choose a vehicle to escape from the weight of your daily routine. Try maintaining your bliss (runner's high) by continuing relaxation techniques immediately after exercising, throughout the day, and at bedtime.

It's time we tried to put the soul, the sensuality, yes, the spirituality back into the fun we have playing at exercise. Getting older—past 40, 50, then 60—happens, and aging is relentless. We can't neglect the playfulness of healthy recreation. Such a perspective could bring us closer to our own spirituality as we shed our ties and sport coats and strip down to the basics several times a week in an effort to either get or stay fit over 40.

Don't think about it.

Just do it.

Glossary

"Abs": Thick row of muscles covering the abdomen, which are separated into several envelopes of muscle tissue.

ACSM: American College of Sports Medicine.

Adultery: Being at the right place at the right time with the wrong woman.

Aerobic exercise: What running, biking, cross-country skiing, and swimming are all about. The object is to work the heart and lungs.

Alcoholic: (1) Someone who drinks more than his or her doctor. (2) Someone who drinks just as much as you and me but doesn't act nice. (3) Someone who lets alcohol interfere with his or her life. (4) Someone who lets alcohol interfere with another person's life.

Alcoholism: The hereditary chemical, mental, or physical addiction to alcohol.

Alzheimer's disease: An inexorable destruction of brain cells showing no preference for rich or poor, professional or laborer; characterized by a specific change in the appearance of brain cells leading to mental deterioration.

Amylase: The mouth enzyme that breaks down everyday starches in the mouth, allowing bacteria to have a field day, eventually producing cavities in those wide cracks left behind. Also, the pancreatic hormone responsible for breaking down starches in the gut, where it is secreted.

Android alopecia: Typical temporal balding paradoxically due to more than adequate amounts of the male hormone testosterone.

Anaerobic threshold: This is that painful point at which the buildup of CO_2 and lactate in the muscles surpasses available oxygen. It's when the muscles burn and the body begins to beg for mercy.

Anemia: Any hemoglobin less than 13 or 14 mg% in a man. Such a discovery warrants assessment of red cell size and coloring. Small size and light color suggest iron deficiency. Large size and dark coloring indicate folate or B$_{12}$ deficiency. Each type of abnormality warrants appropriate action to rule out iron deficiency anemia, folate deficiency, or vitamin B$_{12}$ deficiency.

Angina: Chest pain attributed to coronary artery narrowing due to actual arteriosclerosis or spasm. Typically, such pain is over the front of the chest ("Doc, it's like being pinned by a truck!"), radiating to the cheek or, frequently, down the left arm.

Antioxidants: Vitamins such as A, beta carotene (found in broccoli, brussels sprouts, and cauliflower), C, selenium, BHA, BHT, and possibly chromium. These vitamins are supposed to speed recovery and prevent cancer.

Anxiety: An almost palpable, painful perception of tension and apprehension, coupled with increased autonomic nervous system activity, rapid heartbeat, flushing, and sweating.

Arrhythmia: Any irregular heart beat or rhythm. This potentially serious event can run the gamut from benign, or safe—i.e., one that's just plain irregular—to atrial flutter or fibrillation that can raise a doctor's eyebrows. The real villains are ventricular fibrillation or tachycardia. These are the times that test any first responder's mettle.

Arteriosclerosis: When calcium and fibrous plaques are deposited in the blood vessels. The process is exacerbated by high cholesterol, especially the LDL and VLDL varieties. Other major causes include smoking and hypertension.

Arthritis: Painful swelling and inflammation of any of several joints in the body. Symmetric or asymmetric, arthritis can usually be controlled with an anti-inflammatory medication.

Asthma: So-called small-airway disease, when muscular smaller airways react or go into spasm either because of an intrinsic genetic factor or an extrinsic antagonist such as exercise, cold, allergies, or any of a myriad of pollutants.

Atherosclerosis: The buildup of plaques of fat and calcium in the arteries that ultimately clog the arteries, leading to strokes and heart attacks. This process is increased in someone who has hypertension or hypercholesterolemia.

Atopic dermatitis: A dry rash around the edge of the mouth or nose associated with asthma. It usually responds well to topical steroids, which are relatively harmless if used carefully.

Basal cell carcinoma: Similar to squamous carcinomas, found on exposed areas of fair-skinned people. It has a beaded or pearly appearance and can be eradicated with fairly straightforward Moh's or excisional surgery. If in doubt, take it out.

Bicycle stress test: This can be the ideal method of performing a cardiac stress test on anyone who has had a stroke, has rheumatoid or degenerative arthritis of the ankles, knees, or hips, and is unable to run on a treadmill.

Bone mass: The actual weight of calcified bone in the body compared with the other components such as muscle or fat.

Cancer: When normal cells in the body go haywire—that is, they begin growing irregularly and uncontrollably. The incidence of cancer is related to genetic background and exposure to environmental toxins (including too much sun). Cancer may even be viral in etiology. Though cancer is an equal-opportunity destroyer, individuals who avoid certain carcinogens or combinations thereof (like the evil combo of alcohol and smoking) can diminish their risk of contracting the Big C.

Cardiac pacemaker: Either permanent or temporary, external or internal, designed to pace the heart when its own (intrinsic) pacemaker cells are no longer effective.

Cardiac stress test (GXT): An extremely safe, systematic, monitored method of exercising a subject (patient) to ideally at least 85 percent of his or her maximal heart rate. It is the second most basic method (after a resting EKG) for initiating and recording rhythm disturbances, ischemia, or exercise-related chest pain.

Carcinoembryonic antigen (CEA): An antigen found elevated in colon cancer cases. This immunological test is especially convenient for detecting cancer recurrence in someone who has already had a resection of a primary cancer.

CAT scan: A radiographic technique that takes ultrathin and extremely sensitive X-ray pictures of slices of the body, either with or without contrast or barium so that special structures can be successfully delineated.

Cholesterol: Divided into good fat (HDL) and bad fat (LDL), cholesterol is crucial for steroid synthesis and contributes to myelin nerve sheaths and the production of the sex hormones.

Circuit training: Moving from one exercise to another in a set routine used to develop muscular strength or boost aerobic capacity.

Colon: The part of the large intestine from the end of the small bowel (beginning with that nasty little devil, the appendix) and ending at the rectum or anus.

Colonoscopy: A test using a flexible fiber-optic tube that, under trained guidance, can travel the complete large bowel and safely biopsy any polyps or abnormal tissue that happens to be along the way.

Complete protein: Combining complementary vegetable amino acids to produce a protein capable of building muscle mass.

Congestive heart failure: When the heart lacks total ability to adequately pump blood through the aorta to the vital organs of the body. The result can be fluid buildup in the liver, spleen, or legs (right-sided heart failure) or in the lungs (left-sided heart failure). The cause can be from some form of heart dysfunction such as diabetic coronary disease, a cardiac infarction, or a ventricular aneurysm (the heart tissue balloons out instead of pumping functionally).

Crunches: Quick, incomplete sit-ups that bypass stressing the quads on the front of the thighs or hamstrings. This method of strengthening the abdominal muscles (abs) isolates the upper muscles from the lower muscles that fill the rectal sheath.

Dementia: A confused state from reversible or irreversible causes. From the Latin "to be possessed by demons."

Depression: The most common mood disorder (dysphoria). Can be limited to a month or less or can last a lifetime. Treatments include cognitive therapy, antidepressant medications such as tricyclics (Amitriptyline) and serotonin reuptake inhibitors (Prozac, Zoloft, Paxil), and, as a last resort, shock therapy. The ultimate expression of depression is suicide.

Diabetes: An inability to absorb glucose due to inadequate amounts of insulin. Diabetes is frequently associated with high cholesterol, triglyceride, and uric acid levels known as type IV hyperlipoproteinemia. The two types of diabetes are Type 1, or juvenile-onset diabetes, and Type 2, or adult-onset, obesity-related diabetes.

Dipyridamole stress test: Another of the noninvasive tests for coronary and cardiac muscle ischemia. This test is associated with greater risk than the thallium scan due to reactions to dipyridamole.

Diverticula: Small weak spots in the wall of the large bowel that produce little sacs that can become enlarged or easily inflamed. One way to avoid this condition is to stay on a so-called high-residue (high fiber) diet.

Diverticulitis: When diverticuli become inflamed, they produce fever, pain, perforation, sepsis, and even obstruction. This condition can require taking antibiotics and resting the bowel with nasogastric suction.

Duke's A or B cancer of the GI tract: A readily operable cancer of the gastrointestinal tract. Early discovery is the name of the game. Can be detected by checking for blood in the stool (stool guaiacs).

Dysphasia: Difficulty or even painful swallowing.

Dyspareunia: Painful intercourse. (Old medical student saying: "Dis pareunia is better than no pareunia at all.")

Echo stress test: A noninvasive (meaning no needles) method to delineate heart muscle dysfunction associated with ischemia while the patient is exercising at lower than the maximum heart rate. A way to visualize directly poorly functioning cardiac muscle during submaximal exercise.

Eczema: A dry rash of the skin characterized by flaking and itching. It can often respond to steroid anti-inflammatory cream.

EEG: A test showing the electrical activity of the brain. Can indicate increased activity of a seizure disorder or localized diffuse slowing from a mass that may interfere with normal electrical activity.

Ejaculation: The usually pleasurable release of the fluid carrying sperm during intercourse.

Electrical stimulation: A physical therapy technique that electrically activates muscles that may have been injured. Such a repetitive low-level stimulus can help an injured muscle heal by improving blood flow without taxing injured tissue.

Emphysema: A condition that creates breathing difficulties caused by hyperinflation of the lungs, a result of air being trapped by less elastic, less distensible lung tissue. A major cause of emphysema is smoking.

Endocrine glands: A series of organs, including the thyroid, the gonads, and the adrenals, that secrete many of the hormones that regulate most body functions. Most endocrine glands are in a feedback loop with the "master gland," the pituitary, located in the base of the brain.

Endocrinologist: An internist who specializes in the hormones and glands. This physician is an expert in diabetes, calcium problems, and diseases of the thyroid.

Endoscopy: Looking into any of the hollow viscus organs (tubes) of the body with a fiber-optic-lit tube. A trained physician can learn about the stomach (upper endoscopy), the colon (colonoscopy, sigmoidoscopy, or anoscopy), or the trachea (bronchoscopy) this way. Biopsies, cultures, or secretions for cancer cells may also be taken.

Endurance activity: Any activity or exercise that promotes the capacity to sustain while performing continuous submaximal muscle contractions over extended time periods. For example, distance running rather than sprinting. A type of exercise that endures with age.

Esophagus: The flexible conduit of food from the back of the mouth to the stomach. The sphincter at the lower end, if it is functioning properly, successfully prevents reflux that can lead to heartburn or even bleeding.

Exocrine glands: Certain cells in the body that secrete enzymes like those in the pancreas to produce amylase or lipase, which go directly via a duct into the duodenum. Such secretion is directly stimulated by certain substances—in this case, fats.

Fast-twitch fibers: The white fibers that are responsible for short, fast athletic activities, such as sprinting, which predominate in the young athlete.

Fat-soluble vitamins: A, D, E, K. Necessary for the functioning of the body. Because they are stored in fat, they are capable of building up to toxic levels.

Ferritin: A measure of saturation of the iron-binding substance apoferritin. Low serum ferritin indicates iron deficiency anemia. If found in a 40-year-old man, he should have his colon studied from front to back.

Fiber: A necessary, but often lacking, component of a healthy diet. When taken in amounts of 25 to 50 grams per day, fiber prevents diverticular disease, colon cancer, diabetes, and cardiovascular disease, among other diet-related ailments. Foods great for fiber include legumes, oat bran, raisins, and other plant material.

Flexible sigmoidoscopy: A Japanese-invented test using a fiber-optic scope that allows the physician to view the lower gastrointestinal tract from the rectum through the sigmoid and nearly up to the bend at the spleen. Allows the physician to obtain biopsies safely. A test often recommended after blood is found in the stools.

Free fatty acids (FFAs): Fat breakdown products that can be helpful nutritionally when there is a shortage of readily available and efficiently burning carbohydrates. Coffee can mobilize FFAs as well.

Gallbladder disease: Women and female children first. Medical students learn it as the Five Fs (fat, female, flatulent, forty, flaky), but men of the right genetic predisposition can also get this disease.

Gluteus maximus ("glutes"): The strong muscles comprising the buttocks. What you're probably sitting on right now.

Gout: When uric acid crystals collect in the joints. Classically, this ends up being the first joint of the big toe (podagra), but gout can affect other joints such as the ankle or the other toes.

Guaiac test: The original and simple method of looking for hidden blood in the stool.

Hamstrings ("hams"): The muscles at the back of the thigh.

Heartburn: A pain radiating from the chest that can be mistaken for a heart attack. Actually originates in the solar plexus. May have started after eating some kind of gut bomb. Should quickly improve with an antacid such as Maalox or Mylanta. The doctor can try relieving the pain with a "GI cocktail" composed of an antacid, viscus xylocaine, and donnatal (an antispasmodic).

Hemoccult: One of two reliable (sensitive and specific) tests for blood in the gut from any source, ranging from a polyp to a cancer.

Herpes hominis: Characterized as Type 1 (oral) or Type 2 (genital). Either type can reside in the mouth or on the genitals. Usually caused by a virus and spread by sexual contact. Recurrences seem exacerbated by stress. The antiviral medication Zovirax, taken topically or orally, can lessen attacks and be used as prophylaxis.

Herpes zoster (shingles): Caused by a virus similar to the varicella (chicken pox) virus. Attacks the nerve roots, producing a painful constellation of typical vesicles, pain, or radiating postherpetic neuralgia.

Hiatal hernia: A weakness in the area of the diaphragm, usually where the esophagus enters the stomach. Part of the stomach can pass up through the hole, producing pain, especially after too much late-night eating or from just lying flat after eating.

High-density lipoproteins (HDLs): The good guys among the fats. Can be elevated owing to genetic background—i.e., you chose the right parents—or exercise. Elevations in this category tend to lessen cardiac mortality and morbidity.

Hodgkin's disease: One of the lymph node tumors that, in some cases, can be more responsive to treatment. After a diagnostic surgical excisional biopsy, Hodgkin's disease is often treated with radiation or chemotherapy.

Hyperthermia: An elevation in body temperature due to fluid loss from the body. Usually occurs in very hot environments, frequently secondary to dehydration. Even a 5 percent weight loss can lead to hyperthermia. Heat exhaustion occurs at body temperatures of less than 103°F, heat stroke at temperatures over 106°F.

Hypothermia: A decrease in body temperature to well below 98.6°F. Diagnosis may require a special thermometer that drops below 96°F.

Impotence: An inability to achieve or maintain an erection sufficient for sustained and successful vaginal penetration.

Intervals: A near-maximum or maximum-speed workout of a selected distance repetitively (e.g., 400 m, 800 m, or 1,500 m), usually with a slow workout or rest period in between. The best way to train the fast-twitch muscles (white fibers) to tolerate speed.

Intervertebral discs: The cartilaginous cushions separating the vertebrae. These discs are the culprits that become squashed and can extrude to pinch one of the nerve rootlets on their way to the arms or legs, producing pain and possibly muscle weakness.

Intrinsic factor: A vital protein substance secreted by the parietal cells in the stomach for the absorption of dietary vitamin B_{12}.

Irritable colon: Painful spasms of the colon set off by excessive cholinergic discharges. May be associated with diarrhea or even such signs of colitis as mucous or blood.

Isometric exercise: Exercising by keeping a muscle in a fixed position as the tension is increased.

Isokinetic exercise: Exercise designed to develop strength by using maximal force through the full range of motion and at variable speeds. Includes such designer exercise devices as Nautilus or Cybex. Perfect for the busy 40 year old who in midlife has less time for exercise.

Isotonic exercise: Concentric and eccentric contractions against either a constant or variable resistance.

Karvonen formula: A handy way to determine the target heart rate if you are taking a medication that has lowered the baseline heart rate.

Lactase deficiency: The loss in the body of the enzyme lactase, which breaks down milk. Affects Asians, blacks, and whites, in that order.

Laser excision: Currently the most effective, state-of-the-art way to remove skin cancers.

Lesegue's sign: A diagnostic test in which the physician extends the lower leg against the flexed thigh. Useful to test pain at the sciatic notch when the lower lumbar nerve roots are compromised from a protruding intervertebral disc.

Lipase: One of the enzymes secreted by the pancreas that are necessary for fat breakdown and absorption.

Lipids: Water-insoluble fats found in the body. Some are necessary for survival. Too many are a "no-no."

Low-density lipoproteins (LDLs): The bad guys in the fat family. Can be elevated owing to various factors, including obesity, dietary indiscretion, certain medications, or genetic predisposition. LDLs respond to some old and new medications ranging from nicotinic acid to one of the designer medications such as Lovastatin (Mevacor), Pravastatin (Pravachol), or Simvastatin (Zocor).

Lycra: Unisexual pantyhose for the "X" generation to exercise in.

Maximum oxygen uptake: The maximum number of liters of oxygen taken up per kilogram of body weight per minute. This is a measure of just how efficiently the body can use oxygen. Generally, aerobic athletes such as rowers and cross-country skiers have this one sewn up.

Melanoma: A cancer of the pigmented skin cells (melanocytes), perhaps set off by overexposure to UV light. Can be traced to sunburn or repeated sun exposure in childhood. Represents 1 to 2 percent of all cancers. Prognosis is best if the little devil is less than 4 millimeters in diameter at the time of diagnosis.

Midlife: That time in life when the body goes to hell, when friends and family—especially the kids—turn on you, when the boss becomes a capricious slave driver, and when you realize there is less life ahead than behind. Can occur any time between the ages of 30 and 80.

Nitrates: Preservatives in hot dogs and other cured meats that are considered potential carcinogens.

NMR (nuclearmagnetic resonance): Especially good test employing radio magnetic waves to look at soft structures in the body.

Non-seminomateous germ-cell tumors: One of the so-called good actors of the testicular carcinomas. Responds to castration and radical inguinal lymph node resection by a urologist. If already disseminated, can be treated with combination chemotherapy by a compassionate oncologist.

Nonsteroidal anti-inflammatory: A medication other than prednisone with anti-inflammatory properties, yet fewer adverse side effects than a steroid. Best taken with food.

Overflow incontinence: A sudden loss of water through the urinary tract due, for example, to an obstructive prostate. The bladder stretches until the increased back pressure blasts urine out, usually at an inopportune moment.

Overtraining: Training to the point at which the body begins to feel flat, tired, sometimes depressed, and flat out rejects further exercise. Sometimes leads to an elevated pulse in the morning. This is the time to listen to the body and take it easy.

Pace interval: Exercising at race pace to train the body to become comfortable with speed work.

Panic attack: Emotional reaction to various stressors resulting in physiological manifestations such as tachycardia and palpitations, excessive sweating, paranoia, severe anxiety, and fear. Treatable with antianxiety medications and various behavioral therapies.

Penile implants: Implants in the penis of stiff plastic rods or indwelling sacs that can be inflated by hand for intercourse. These may be the only option for someone, such as an advanced diabetic who has neuropathy and impotence.

Peptic ulcer disease: Includes ulcers in the stomach or the duodenum. Certain folks have a tendency to be hypersecreters of stomach acid. Foods such as coffee, chocolate, heavy spices, and alcohol can eliminate the mucus secreted by other cells that would ordinarily serve as a protective barrier against the stomach's own acid.

Percent body fat: A measurement of fat in the body that indicates a certain level of fitness. Generally, the lower the percentage the better. Average figures for the 40 year old, 17 to 23 percent; the 50 year old, 18 to 24 percent; and the 60 year old, 19 to 25 percent. By comparison, an elite male athlete could run 4 to 7 percent body fat and an elite female athlete 12 to 17 percent.

Periodontal disease: The number one dental problem for men over 40. An infection of the gums as well as the supporting tissue of the teeth.

Periodontitis: Infection due to retained bacteria in plaque and cavities under the gums.

Polycose: A long-chain sugar used in sports drinks that enhances absorption of water and provides excellent, if short-term, nutrition.

Polyp: An abnormal growth anywhere in the GI tract having the potential to become malignant and cancerous. Certainly, any found in the colon should be removed either via colonoscopy or surgery. Many polyps have the tendency to show malignant transformation at their bases, something that can be detected by surgical excision.

Prostatism: Prostate enlargement and blockage resulting in urinary frequency (you go a lot), hesitancy (you stand in front of the urinal waiting to go a lot), dysuria (it hurts to go), hematuria (you pee red), and incomplete emptying of the bladder. The worst scenario is urosepsis, when infected urine becomes blood-borne, producing fever, shakes, chills, and possibly death if not treated quickly enough.

Prostatectomy: A urological procedure involving the slicing away of extra or obstructing prostate tissue.

Psoriasis: A rash of protean quality manifesting as satellite (mummular) or grapelike (guttate) clumps of flaking skin usually most visible in the hair line, on the elbows, on the knees, or on the penis.

Psychomotor performance: A combination of cerebral and physical activity required to perform sophisticated movements or activities.

Pulmonary functions: Breathing tests that measure how efficiently the lungs are functioning.

Pyramid system: A method of exercise weight lifting that starts with a set of three to five reps, adding 5 pounds with each new set, and doing three to five sets until the body poops out.

Rectum: The place where processed food exits via the anus; the last sphincter of the GI tract.

Reflux: Often accompanies a hiatal hernia—when stomach acid goes backward up into the esophagus. Ouch!

Reiter's syndrome: The combination of urethritis, conjunctivitis, and arthritis caused in some by a chlamydia vaginal infection from a sexual partner. A more common cause is food poisoning.

Residual volume: The amount of air left in the lungs after a complete expiration.

Resistance exercises: The handy technique of using one's own body weight to strengthen the muscles. This includes such age-old favorites as push-ups, pull-ups, and tummy crunches.

Rest-pause system: Doing maximal weights until exhaustion.

Rheumatic fever: A migratory joint inflammation hitting two or more joints at a time. Responds to a combination of anti-inflammatories and antibiotics.

Rheumatoid arthritis: An acute and chronic inflammatory process involving the wrist and fingers, producing such changes as swan neck deformities of the fingers and ulnar deviation of the hands. This rampant problem responds to anti-inflammatories, gold shots, and sometimes even antineoplastic drugs such as methotrexate or cytoxan.

Sandwich generation: Those members of society squeezed between hormonally challenged children and deteriorating parents.

Sciatic notch: The primary passageway of the lower lumbar nerve roots through the main butt muscle (the gluteus maximus) to the legs.

Set system: A given number of repeat exercises (e.g., 10 to 15), resting, then repeating. The super set system means working opposing antagonist exercises.

Slow-twitch fibers: Red fibers responsible for aerobic or long-distance training.

Squamous cell carcinoma: A flat and scaling skin lesion found often on sun-exposed areas of the skin, sometimes resulting from earlier excessive sun exposure. Easily removed with excisional biopsy and pathological confirmation of complete removal.

Stretching: The process of actively yet slowly pulling the muscles out to near-maximal length. If done properly, a way to enjoy exercising more and avoid injuries. Stretches should be static, not jerky, and should be maintained from 8 to 15 seconds.

Super circuit system: Combines peripheral heart action, sets, and circuit training systems. The secret is light weights and high reps while exercising alternate muscle groups.

Terminal insomnia: When an individual has no trouble falling asleep but repeatedly awakens in the early hours of the morning. Often characterizes depression.

Testosterone: One of the several male sex hormones secreted by the testes and responsible for secondary sexual characteristics such as a deep voice, facial hair, and much of the sex drive.

Thallium stress test: A test in which radioactive thallium is systematically taken up by the heart muscle. The test is used specifically to view actual heart muscle dysfunction resulting from ischemia due to inadequate coronary blood supply.

Thrombophlebitis: Vein inflammation. A condition that warrants no-nonsense intervention if it includes one of the major leg veins, such as the femoral. Thrombophlebitis has the tendency to produce and send blood clots known as pulmonary emboli the lungs. Treatment includes heat, elevation, and anticoagulation with Heparin and then Coumadin.

Trapezius ("traps"): The strong muscles running from the back of the skull onto the shoulders. These muscles support the head and can be injured in typical whiplash accidents.

Triglycerides: One of the lipoproteins often elevated in the Type 4 hyperlipoproteinemia individual—that is, someone who is running a high glucose count, especially if he or she is developing late-onset or maturity-onset diabetes. Individuals who have elevated triglyceride counts also tend to run high uric acid levels and have bouts of gout. Treatment includes a low-fat diet or certain medications such as Clofibrate (Atromid), or Gemfibrozil (Lopid), or niacin (Nicolar).

Type 1 diabetes: Sometimes called juvenile-onset diabetes. Onset usually occurs under the age of 20. Associated with diabetic ketoacidosis and other dangerous metabolic imbalances.

Type 2 diabetes: Genetic, one of insulin paucity or deficiency rather than insulin deficit. Onset is a function of obesity or age.

Ultrasound: Low-intensity waves that can massage muscles at a microscopic level.

Urethritis: Inflammation of the lower portion of the water tube, causing burning and/or a yellow discharge. Offending organisms can range from chlamydia, trichomonas, gonorrhea, or the most frequent offender, a nonspecific urethritis, possibly viral in etiology. If your sex partner has it, so could you. If you think you might have urethritis, get a culture, as there are some effective medications (such as the tetracyclines or the penicillins) that can adequately treat the problem.

Urinary frequency: Aka "peeing a lot," either during the day or at night (nocturia). Causes range from urinary tract infection (UTI) and diabetes to functional (meaning, it's a head thing) or just drinking too much coffee or beer.

Urologist: A doctor who specializes in taking care of the genitourinary tract—including kidney stones or cancer, the ureters and urethra, prostate, penis, and testicles.

VO_{max}: The maximal number of milliliters of oxygen the body can metabolize per kilogram per minute.

Water-soluble vitamins: C, thiamine, riboflavin, niacin, folic acid, B_{12}, biotin, pantothenic acid. These vitamins dissolve easily in water and can be excreted through the urinary tract.

Ventilation perfusion ratio: Just how much air the body can bring in to exchange with the blood that passes through the alveoli or smallest air spaces in the lungs.

Vital capacity: The amount of air the body can force out of the lungs after a maximal inspiration.

Index